# Bills of Hea

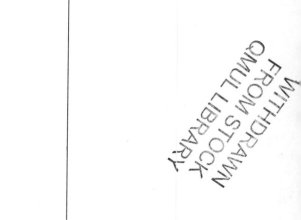

# Bills of Health

Richard Lawson
MBBS, MRCPsych.

Foreword by
Jonathon Porritt

Radcliffe Medical Press

Oxford and New York

©1997 Richard Lawson

Radcliffe Medical Press Ltd
18 Marcham Road, Abingdon, Oxon OX14 1AA, UK

Radcliffe Medical Press, Inc.
141 Fifth Avenue, New York, NY 10010, USA

British Library Cataloguing in Publication Data

A catalogue record for this book is available from the British Library.

ISBN    1 85775 101 9

Library of Congress Cataloging-in-Publication Data

Lawson, Richard, 1946–
    Bills of health / Richard Lawson.
       p. cm.
    Includes bibliographical references and index.
    ISBN 1–85775–101–9
    1. Public health–Social aspects–Great Britain.   2. Public
health–Economic aspects–Great Britain.   3. Public health–
Environmental aspects–Great Britain.   4. Medical policy–Great
Britain.   5. Health promotion–Government policy–Great Britain.
6. Great Britain–Social conditions.   7. Great Britain–Economic
conditions.   8. Great Britain–Environmental conditions.   I. Title.
RA485.L37     1996
362.1′0941–dc20     96–13782
                      CIP

Typeset by EXPO Holdings, Malaysia
Printed and bound by Redwood Books, Trowbridge, Wiltshire

147759
M

This book is respectfully dedicated to the next
Minister of Public Health

# Contents

# Foreword

*Bills of Health* sets the ongoing debate about funding within the National Health Service in its proper context. When our very way of life depends on undermining people's health, in body, mind and spirit, it is hardly surprising that we find it harder and harder to pay the bills at the end of each year. It is not the National Health Service which is unsustainable, but our idiotic accounting practices and perverse notions of progress and standard of living.

Jonathon Porritt
*August 1996*

# Preface

This book examines the impact of external conditions – unemployment, poverty, social and environmental conditions – on the health of the population and measures their effect, so far as is possible, on spending within the British National Health Service. It is intended for all readers who are interested in matters of health, politics, social conditions and the environment. It is hoped that it will be of especial interest to health workers, medical and nursing students; supplying vital background data to their health care studies. It does not attempt to be a definitive scientific textbook, but hopes to map a territory and preliminary method, to which future academic work will add detail.

Richard Lawson
*August 1996*

# Acknowledgements

Grateful thanks for help and encouragement go to the following.

- Nicky, Joe, Freya and Laurie for tolerating my mental and physical absence over the past year.

- Dr Peter Ambrose; Brenda Boardman; Ann Boyle; Tim Brown; Bob Chew at OHE; Andy Cunningham; Peter Grainger; David Gunnell; Keith Horton; Dr Martin Hartog; Philip Insall of Sustrans; Ray Ilsley; Colin Kirkby; David Leadbetter; Rita Miller; Andy Moore; Peter Phillimore; Diane Smithson at Weston General Hospital library; Graham Schipp; Pete Stockwell; Chris Tranter; Professor Richard Wilkinson. Many helpful librarians and government officials. My friends, family and colleagues in the Green Party and the Green movement generally for help, support and inspiration.

My apologies and thanks go to the many other unnamed workers who helped me along the way.

Many of the figures are reproduced with the permission of the Controller of HMSO.

The policies put forward in this book are not necessarily official policies of the Green Party.

While acknowledging the help given by the above, the responsibility for any errors in this book rests entirely with myself.

# Introduction

There is more to healthy living than brown bread and jogging. Changes in personal habits are undoubtedly important, but they are limited by external conditions – for instance, low-fat, high-fibre joggers may do themselves more harm than good by exercising on days when traffic pollution has created poor air quality. Real health demands political, economic, social and environmental changes.

In July 1992, the government introduced the Health of the Nation programme, which sets targets for improvements in five key areas of health: coronary heart disease and stroke, cancer, mental illness, HIV/AIDS and accidents.

At the beginning of the Health of the Nation consultation process, William Waldegrave, the then Secretary of State for Health, recognized the role of his office in 'causing reforms in other government departments that would improve health'. Success, he said, will come through public policies, by policy makers at all levels considering the health dimension when debating policies, with the aim of improving and maintaining health, not simply health care.

In the same vein Virginia Bottomley, the next Secretary of State for Health, emphasized in her introduction to the Health of the Nation White Paper that the pursuit of 'health' in its widest sense was not just the responsibility of the Department of Health: 'there is a commitment to the pursuit of "health" in its widest sense, both within Government and beyond. Within Government this reflects not only my role as Secretary of State for Health but also the responsibilities of my colleagues in other Departments.[1]

Clearly, then, at the heart of this exercise there is a recognition of the fact that there is more to health than handing out pills and providing hospital beds, and that public health is the responsibility of public policy. The buzzword is 'intersectoral' thinking, whereby employment, housing, industry, transport and welfare policies are developed with public health in mind. However, the perception of those toiling at the sharp end of the delivery of health care is that the responsibility for improving the nation's health – health promotion – has fallen fair and square on to their shoulders. Health promotion tasks mean that doctors and nurses are to weigh, measure and record lifestyle habits such as smoking, drinking, diet and exercise. Although this is widely seen as a worthy exercise by the public, general practitioners (GPs) and primary health care teams are less than enthusiastic for three reasons. First, they are having difficulty in meeting the demands of the core duty of diagnosing and treating ailments of all kinds from colds to cancer, at a time when the support that primary care expects of hospital services is severely constrained by waiting lists of varying lengths from the embarrassing to the surreal. Second, British physicians are not convinced that there is good scientific evidence that 'health check-ups' actually do anyone any good. The *British Medical Journal* (*BMJ*) in April 1995 published papers suggesting that health checks for unselected middle-aged people achieve little or no reduction in smoking or excessive drinking, and that intensive group health education offers little benefit over standard GP advice to reduce fat, increase exercise and stop smoking. Those who take up the offer to visit the doctor for a health check are usually the middle class 'worried well' rather than the low-waged, unskilled and unemployed people whose health is mainly at risk. Third, it is unanimously believed that if government wishes to reduce smoking-related diseases such as lung cancer and coronary heart disease then tobacco advertising should be banned, but this is something that the government is singularly reluctant to do. The net result is that health care workers feel that they are being required to make bricks without straw.

The contribution of public policy to public health may well begin with the elimination of tobacco advertising, but by no means does it end there. Unemployment, poverty, poor housing, stress and environmental pollution are all known to have an impact on human health. A large amount of scientific work exists on these subjects, but little of this reaches the general public.

The laws of supply and demand bear heavily on the NHS. Although it receives an extra 1% or 2% of its annual budget here and there, the health service budget is cash limited, whereas the conditions that cause ill-health seem to be unlimited. At its inception, it was argued that access to free health care would result in a healthier population and therefore demand for NHS services would be self-limiting or even diminishing. Half a century later, this optimism is seen to be unfounded, and the received wisdom is that demand for health care is infinite: the more services are available, the more people will wish to use them. Rationing, whether explicit or implicit, is seen as the only realistic possibility. Private health care is growing, while the NHS services are rationed by the length of a waiting list, although, at the same time attempts are being made to shorten lists by statistically massaging them and demanding ever more productivity from medical and nursing staff. This is causing chronic stress in clinical staff to the extent that in some cases clinical efficiency is now dangerously impaired.[2] An Australian[3] study found that 0.8% of people (25 000–30 000) admitted to hospitals suffered preventable adverse events leading to permanent disability and 14 000 (0.5%) died. Stress in the NHS is probably worse in the UK than in Australia, and the casualty rate is probably therefore worse. Any measure that removes stress from the health services will lead to significant gains in safety.

One of the results of this situation is a perennial complaint from health care workers that the NHS is underfunded, which is met by a barrage of statistics from the Health Secretary to the effect that NHS spending is going up in real terms. Both are right. Spending has been going up, although much of the spending has been consumed by the huge administrative costs of the health service reforms in the late 1980s. In 1992, the NHS central management bill doubled as its staff numbers increased by 1800. In a parliamentary answer to Alan Milburn MP in June 1995 figures were obtained for administration costs for regional and district health authorities:

| Year | Cost |
|---|---|
| 1991–92 | £775 400 000 |
| 1993–94 | £1 045 100 000 |

This represents a 35% cost increase

The funding of the UK NHS fares badly by almost all international comparisons. In 1990, among the 21 member countries of the Organization for Economic Co-operation and Development (OECD) the UK was fifth from the bottom on total health expenditure per person, third from bottom on real (adjusted by the consumer price index) total health expenditure per person and bottom for total health expenditure as a percentage of GDP at market prices.

The NHS budget is planned to increase by 0.5% annually, and increased demands by an ageing population and increased costs owing to improvements in medical technology reduce this by 1% annually, so that the budget is falling behind by half a percentage point annually. Increased administration costs referred to previously further increase the shortfall. Add to this the increased demands created by the conditions considered in this book and the conclusion is that the NHS budget is falling behind significantly year by year.

For this reason, it is imperative in the name of health that combined political pressure from health professionals and voters creates the political will to examine the impact on health (and therefore on the NHS) of adverse social, economic and environmental conditions. It will be found not only that these conditions combine to increase demand on the NHS, but also that measures aimed at rectifying these problems result in savings for the NHS and thus for the whole economy.

This book presents health-related social and ecological research in a way that is accessible to the reader. Its main thrust is to show that policies aimed at improving the health of the nation are cost-effective. This work cannot claim in any way to be scientific or academic; since to produce a credible cost–benefit analysis at that level would take many lifetimes' full effort. Sometimes, fairly crude 'guesstimates' and assumptions have been used to try to give a numerical and financial value to the processes that are being discussed, based on the simple certainty that every aspect of health, right down to the act of sneezing into a paper handkerchief, must have a finite cost. The costs found here vary from detailed figures lifted from respected work to rough assumptions, which have invariably been on the conservative side. It is to be hoped that, in time, careful scientific and actuarial work will firm up the assumptions and 'guesstimates'.

This book covers the impact of external conditions on the health of the nation. The impact of health care delivery, health service structure and administration and the potential for public education to improve the nation's health have purposely been avoided in order to impose some manageability on a vast subject.

Some readers may find the process of assigning financial value to health and disease repugnant. This is understandable. From the viewpoint of the human spirit, health transcends wealth in the same way that a living flower transcends the letters f-l-o-w-e-r and, in the end, ill-health and suffering can never adequately be represented by financial calculations. However, we live in a material world – some would say an excessively materialistic world – in which it is the fashion to count the monetary value of everything. This is tedious, but if it is what it takes to make real improvements in the real health of real people then time spent in counting abstract figures is spent well.

# REFERENCES

1  *The Health of the Nation: A Strategy for Health in England* (1986) (Cm 1986). HMSO, London.

2  Caplan R P (1994) Stress, anxiety and depression in hospital consultants, general practitioners and senior health service managers. *BMJ*: **309**; 1261–3.

3  Australian hospital care study (1995) *New Sci* (10 June): **146**; 5.

# 1

# What makes people ill?

## INTRODUCTION

Pre-war medical students were taught to repeat the mnemonic 'trauma, tumour, tubercle, inflammation, stone' when seeking the cause of any disorder with which they might be confronted. Since then, knowledge has expanded somewhat, but the principle is the same: although disease is infinitely complex in its manifestations, there are only a finite number of processes that can give rise to it. One possible classification recognizes 13 categories of disease process, eight of which, by happy chance, begin with an 'I':

- inborn
- irritation
- infection
- infestation
- immunological
- injury
- inadequate diet
- neoplasia
- endocrine
- degenerative
- psychogenic
- iatrogenic
- pharmacogenic.

Nearly all of these causes are affected by environmental changes, and in most cases these changes are turning out for the worse.

## Inborn (genetic) causes

### Familial diseases

Some diseases are inherited genetically, for example Huntington's chorea and cystic fibrosis. Although they are rare, about 4000 of these familial conditions are recognized. Their effects can range from the mild to the severe. It could be said that they are the only diseases that occur irrespective of any environmental influence, depending entirely on the hand of genetic cards that are dealt to the individual.

## Genetic influence on disease

Aside from overt genetic disease, the genetic hand of cards that we are dealt at conception has an influence on every aspect of our biological existence, including our reaction to psychosocial situations and environmental agents. Some geneticists are claiming that all our actions are predetermined by our genes. This is a minority view with logic that leads to a form of genetic fatalism in which the only hope of real change would come from the molecular scissors and glue wielded by genetic scientists. Since, in their view, the majority who take a balanced stance on the nature–nurture debate are pre-programmed to take that position and the geneticists are likewise locked into their opinions, there is no point in debating the point since change through talking is out of the question.

The practical point to emerge from consideration of genetic influence is that within a broad population there may be a subset who react differently because of their genes. For instance, some people have a deficiency of the enzyme cholinesterase, which makes them extra-sensitive to the action of organophosphorus insecticides. Safety levels which work (relatively speaking) for the general population may be dangerously high for this subgroup. Similarly, epidemiological studies of health influences may not detect severe illnesses caused by an agent in such a genetic subgroup.

## Genetic damage

Radiation and certain chemicals are known to cause mutations (changes) in the genes of the developing embryo with resulting effects in the body – for instance the stunted limbs of children born to mothers who had taken the drug thalidomide. Down's syndrome has been associated with increased radiation dose from natural sources in Kerala (although not in a similarly high natural background in Espirito Santo, Brazil) and from man-made radiation associated with:

- the 1957 Windscale (Sellafield) fire
- Maryport, 16 miles from Sellafield
- at some sites within reach of the Three Mile Island accident.[1]

# Irritation

Acids, alkalis and a variety of other chemicals can damage or kill cells with which they come in contact. This was probably the mode of action of the chemical released at Bhopal.

## Infection

In rising order of size and complexity, infecting agents are: viruses, bacteria, fungi and protozoa. All can cause illnesses ranging from the mild to the fatal. The factors that determine whether an individual will become ill are divided between the host and the environment. Host factors include whether the person is well nourished and coping with stress. Mediating circumstances in the environment include the humidity and quality of the surrounding air and the number and proximity of new people in the person's immediate vicinity.

## Infestation

Complex organisms such as worms and arachnids have adapted themselves to use the human body as their ecological niche. Again, their effects can range from the irritating to the deadly. Some have evolved complex life cycles involving vector (carrier) species. The best-known ecological threat from this source in the UK is the risk of children contracting toxocariasis, a worm infestation, from dog faeces in play areas. Infestation can result in a blind child, however this is fortunately a rare occurrence.

## Immunological

The immune system is the interface between our biological selves and the environment. It distinguishes between 'self-cells' and neutral substances, both of which are to be left alone; and threats such as viruses, bacteria, fungi, protozoa and parasites, which are to be dealt with efficiently. A century ago there were some 150 chemicals in the immediate environment of the average person. Now that number has swollen to 70 000. This is a huge change in our ecological niche over four generations, and presents a significant challenge to our immune systems. In Chapter 8 we will see that there is evidence that our immune systems are beginning to show signs of strain.

## Injury

The capacity for injury to occur has always been with us, but the advent of machinery has magnified the risk. The motor car kills 5000 people on the roads in the UK every year, and injures ten times as many, and the UK has a very good safety record compared with other countries. Speed is directly proportional to the severity of accidents, and lower speed limits, which can now be enforced by video technology, could reduce the number and severity of accidents significantly.

## Inadequate diet

Malnutrition is a common cause of disease in the developing world, and it is a common belief among authorities that it is not a problem in the UK. However, there is evidence that an inadequate diet is a problem for the increasing number of poor in the UK. Even in the well nourished, the amount of additives, pesticides and pollutants present in food may be diminishing our health.

Nutrition affects energy and efficiency of the organism. Improvement in diet, together with better housing and sanitation, is the probable cause of the increase in general health that we have enjoyed since the Second World War. However, there are some flies in this soup of improvement. The quality of food is not best designed for health. It frequently contains too much sugar and fat and not enough fibre, minerals and vitamins. This imbalance is especially pronounced in the poorest 20% of the population. Moreover, sources of food are not as secure as imagined. Sixty per cent of the food we eat is imported, and some of this is from countries that have widespread malnutrition but are forced to export food to repay foreign debt. If there were a general world movement to repudiate these debts, we might see these imports dry up and would then be hard pressed to meet the food needs of the UK population.

## Neoplasia

Neoplasia (new growth) is the general term for cancer, and includes carcinomas, sarcomas and blood conditions such as leukaemia. Death from cancers is rising, as is the number of environmental agents that can cause cancer: radiation and chemicals. The nuclear weapons tests in the 1950s caused innumerable cancer deaths worldwide, and radiation from the Chernobyl accident is estimated potentially to be able to cause a maximum of 250 000 deaths from cancer. Great though this number is, statistics must always be kept in proportion, and the number is a small proportion of the total number of cancer deaths occurring worldwide. Nevertheless, a large proportion of these deaths would not have occurred without the release of radiation, and each case imposes a huge burden on the sufferers and families, and a different kind of burden on the health services. Death from cancers is increasing, and this increase cannot be explained by the increasing age of the population alone.

Many chemicals, both industrial and those in our everyday environment, cause cancer and among the 2000 new chemicals introduced each year there are likely to be one or two that will cause a certain number of cancers in the future.

Recently, Kinlen[2] has accumulated evidence to support the hypothesis that an influx of workers into an area brings with it new infections, which results in extra cases of leukaemia in the local children. This evidence is interesting, but it must be emphasized that no infective agent that can cause leukaemia in humans has been identified, although it is known in cats. If the theory gains ground, we must be prepared to accept that large construction projects must carry with them a burden of increased childhood leukaemias.

## Endocrine

Disorders of some of the glands that regulate the internal environment and processes of the body – pituitary, thyroid, parathyroid, thymus, pancreas, adrenals and gonads – are increasing. Obesity is on the increase, and with it diabetes. One of the clearest sets of evidence relates to the sex hormones, with decreasing sperm count, feminization of embryos and increasing rates of tumours of sex hormone glands being widely reported.

## Degenerative

'Degenerative' disease is a rather miscellaneous category of conditions that covers common arthritis (osteoarthritis) and the effects of ageing. Recently there has been growing interest in 'free radicals' in the causation of some of these problems. These are electrically charged atoms and molecules such as oxgyen (O) atoms and hydroxyl (OH) molecules. They are extremely reactive, and will join to and alter complex cellular structures, leading to cell disorder or death. They are implicated in the causation of some carcinomas and cholesterol plaques. Radiation and some forms of pollution can cause increases in free radicals.

## Psychogenic

The state of our emotions and moods is the final result of many influences – our early upbringing, more recent traumatic experiences, our current situation in life (love life, social life, work life and financial situation), our current state of physical health and the presence of environmental agents such as solvents and perfumes. Although there are an infinite number of causes, and an infinite number of specific states of emotion, they can be classified into four main states: anxiety/stress, anger, depression and euphoria. In addition to these common states which we all experience daily in a minor way, there are two more major complex reaction states – somatization (or functional disorder) and psychosis. The prevalence of these conditions in society is reflected in the number of prescriptions for psychoactive drugs written by doctors, which is showing an upward trend. Clearly, we are operating outside of our design envelope. We were designed to gather foods, to hunt our food in the savannah and occasionally to put up with a brush with the odd sabre-toothed tiger. All of this was good simple fun, to be rounded off in the evening with a tribal dance, perhaps a bit of singing and story-telling, and so to bed. We were not designed to cope with the complexities of modern life, its speed, its information overload, its excesses of sensory input and gratification, its injustices and its machinery.

## Iatrogenic

Much illness with which doctors cope is caused by side-effects of treatments given earlier. To a certain extent, the more medicine that is practised, the more medicine will have to be practised. The longer we keep people alive, the older they get and the more treatment they will need. Viewed from a strictly biological standpoint, medicine is working against the evolutionary pressure of natural selection, so that by keeping alive people who would otherwise have died, and enabling them to reproduce, the general health of the population will gradually diminish. Having recognized this, it is important to stress the right of an individual to receive medical care must ethically always override Darwinian theory.

## Pharmacogenic

Drugs, both licit and illicit, create their own health problems. The use of illicit hard drugs is exploding in cities, and with it robbery to pay for fresh supplies, with consequent treatments for the physically and emotionally traumatized victims of the robbery. Drug abuse also causes numerous diseases, for example abscesses, hepatitis and AIDS, and large amounts of GP time are spent in assessing whether patients have really lost their last prescription or whether they are 'trying it on'.

## IS ILLNESS ON THE INCREASE?

Demand on health services is certainly increasing year by year, but this in itself is no proof that people are becoming iller. It may be that the health services are offering more services, or that patients (aided and abetted by the Patient's Charter) are becoming more demanding. Or it may be both of these things plus the fact that some or all of the population is becoming less healthy. Statistic analyses can help us understand by acting as indices – pointers – to health.

Mortality (death) rates for the UK, as for many other countries, are falling; people are living longer. However, the rate of fall has decreased over the last decade. This decrease in health gain is related to social, economic and environmental conditions. Death rates are falling more slowly in the poorest fractions of society, and for some conditions, for instance coronary heart disease and female lung cancer, the rates are actually increasing in manual classes (Figure 1.1).

Mortality rates are a crude index of real health. It is a simple matter for doctors to treat pneumonia in the elderly with antibiotics, thereby extending life and keeping down the mortality rate, but this activity does not necessarily increase the health of the population, only its age. Years of life are meaningless if they are

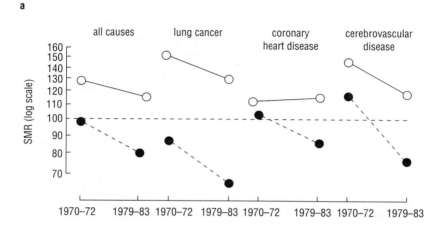

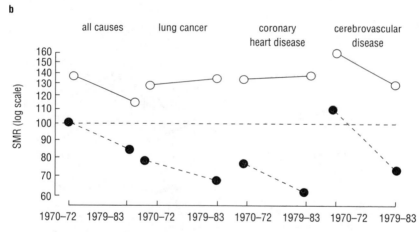

**Figure 1.1**   The increasing differential in mortality between manual and non-manual classes: standardized mortality ratios (SMRs) for select causes of death in Great Britain 1970–72 and 1979–83 for manual (○) and non-manual (●) groups. For each cause and each sex, the overall standardized mortality ratio is 100 in 1979–83. **a** Men aged 20–64. **b** Married women aged 20–54 classified by husband's occupation. Reproduced with permission from Marmot and McDowall.[3]

riddled with illness, pain and disability. To make some kind of measurement of the health of the population, more sophisticated indices are required. Quality adjusted life years (QALYs) and disability adjusted life years (DALYs) have been used to make these measurements. Conditions such as schizophrenia, which have little or no impact on mortality rates, have a large impact on DALYs and therefore on the calls on the NHS.

Figures from the General Household Survey for the years 1962, 1972 and 1988 are set out in Table 1.1. They show a significant increase in longstanding illness.

Figure 1.2 shows the steady increase in the percentage of the population reporting longstanding illness. It shows that the average proportion of those reporting such a condition has increased from 25% to 34% over 15 years.

The main growth areas in longstanding illness are shown in Table 1.2.

**Table 1.1**  Measures of illness

|  | 1962 | 1972 | 1988 |
|---|---|---|---|
| Percentage reporting longstanding illness |  | 22 | 33 |
| No. of prescriptions issued per capita | 4.7 |  | 7.5 |
| Percentage who had been ill in last two weeks |  | 8 | 14 |
| Sickness benefit days/worker | 8.8 |  | 12.2 |

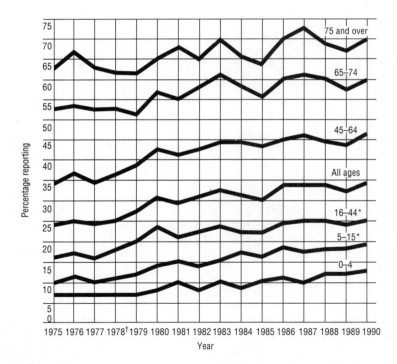

**Figure 1.2**  Percentage of persons reporting longstanding illness by age, Great Britain. *From 1975 to 1978, figures relate to age groups 5–14 and 15–44. †Figures not available in 1978. Reproduced with permission from General Household Survey, OPCS.

**Table 1.2**   Growth areas in longstanding illness

| Condition | No. of sufferers per 1000 |
|---|---|
| Musculoskeletal system | 115 |
| Heart and circulatory | 73 |
| Respiratory system | 67 |
| Digestive system | 32 |
| Nervous system | 24 |
| Eye complaints | 21 |
| Ear complaints | 21 |
| Endocrine and metabolic | 24 |
| Mental disorders | 17 |
| Skin complaints | 16 |
| Genitourinary system | 13 |
| Neoplasms and benign growths | 8 |
| Blood and related organs | 4 |
| Infectious disease | 2 |

It is well known of course, that asthma is increasing in prevalence (chapter 12), as are other forms of allergy. Conditions related to intolerance of foods and other substances – migraine and irritable bowel syndrome – are increasing in prevalence.

It is therefore apparent that, for a variety of reasons, demand on the health service is increasing, and that one of the reasons is that people are experiencing more ill-health. The increased demand for health care is outstripping the supply, so that although it is true that more resources in real terms are being put into the NHS, real waiting lists (as opposed to redefined waiting lists) are getting longer, treatment is becoming more rushed, complaints against doctors are increasing and staff morale is deteriorating.

# CONCLUSION

The conclusion is that in every way that disease may be caused the general trend indicates that our health will come off worst. Increasing ill-health means increasing demand on the NHS, which in a cash-limited NHS amounts to the same thing as cuts in services. This is why, although the government has indeed been increasing NHS budgets, the perception of NHS users and staff alike – and indeed the evidence of unmassaged figures – is that the NHS is slowly but surely failing to keep up. On the other hand, rectification of the external conditions that are causing health problems could relieve pressure on the NHS so that, without extra spending, the quality of medical care could improve.

# REFERENCES

1    Bertell R (1985) *No Immediate Danger.* The Women's Press, London.

2    Kinlen L J, Dickson M and Stiller C A (1995) Childhood leukemia and non-Hodgkin lymphoma near large rural construction sites, with a comparison with the Sellafield nuclear site. *BMJ.* **310**; 163–8.

3    Marmot M G and McDowall M E (1986) Mortality decline and widening social inequalities. *Lancet.* **28**; 274–6.

# 2

# The impact of unemployment on health

## INTRODUCTION

There is no reasonable doubt that the health of unemployed people is worse than the health of those who have employment. The debate has moved on to the question of the extent to which unemployment directly causes people to become ill, and to what extent this observed ill-health is due to the fact that those who are often sick are more likely to lose their jobs. Research has shown that the latter effect is not enough to account for all the sickness that is observed.[1]

Another debate mulls over the extent to which it is the poverty associated with unemployment that causes the illness. This debate, although no doubt interesting to the participants, is academic and abstract. From the practical point of view, if in curing unemployment we cure poverty and the health of the people improves as a general result, the objective will have been met.

There is evidence that the long-term unemployed show increased levels of the following:

- mortality
- general practice consultations
- smoking and alcohol consumption
- weight gain and physical inactivity
- mental ill-health
- parasuicide (i.e. suicide attempts)
- suicide
- illicit drug taking.

# MORTALITY AND UNEMPLOYMENT

The mortality rate (the number of deaths for a given number of population) is a crude but useful general indicator of the health of a population. It is a convenient statistic because it can be calculated easily from existing data and it is correlated with other, more accurate, indices of health. For instance, Townsend et al.[2] have shown that the mortality rate for a population correlates with the rates for infant mortality, permanent sickness and disability and the incidence of low birth rate. Mortality rates are therefore useful as long as we bear in mind that they are an indicator, and only indirectly relate to pain, mental illness and minor illnesses.

Brenner[3–7] made a series of studies of mortality (death) rates in the following countries:

- USA between 1909 and 1976
- England and Wales between 1936 and 1976
- England, Wales and Scotland between 1954 and 1976.

After controlling for other factors, he found that national mortality rates were significantly associated with earlier unemployment levels.

Gravelle et al.[8] criticized Brenner's work on the grounds that he could not exclude general poverty problems as causes of the mortality. Other critics pointed out that a time delay is to be expected between becoming unemployed and suffering harm as a result.

Moser et al.[9] therefore studied OPCS (UK Office of Population Census and Surveys) data and related health changes between 1971 and 1981, comparing those who were employed in April 1971 with those who were unemployed. He found that the mortality rate for the unemployed was 36% higher. When the influence of low social class was removed from the figures, the excess fell to 21%.

Gravelle[10] then suggested that this excess might have been due to pre-existent ill-health. Moser then removed from the numbers those who were sick; he also controlled for factors such as housing tenure (tenant/owner-occupier), region of residence and marital state. He still found increased mortality for the unemployed, especially for death from suicide, lung cancer and ischaemic heart disease. He also found that the wives of unemployed men suffered higher mortality than wives of employed men.

## The cost of excess mortality

The conclusion is that, if a person is unemployed, they are more likely to die early. It is possible to quantify this risk. Brenner estimated that unemployment in Great

Britain is associated with tens of thousands of premature deaths. Alex Scott-Samuel[11] used Moser's figures to calculate that, for every 2000 men seeking work, 1.94 of them, and 0.98 of their wives, will die each year as a result of unemployment.

It is therefore possible to work out the number who died in 1993 as a result of unemployment. Taking the unemployment unit (UU) index figure for late 1993 of 3 985 000 unemployed persons, and a female–male ratio of 1:5.7, the number of unemployed men can be calculated to be 3 390 224. The number of men to die in 1993 as a result of unemployment is therefore:

$$\frac{3\ 390\ 224}{2000} \times 1.94 = 3289$$

In 1989 76% of households were formed by couples. To be conservative, let us assume that only 50% of unemployed men are married. The number of wives of unemployed men at risk would therefore be:

$$\frac{3\ 390\ 224}{2 \times 2000} \times 0.98 = 831$$

The total annual death rate due to unemployment is therefore

$$3289 + 831 = 4120$$

The official UK figure for extra costs to the state for one early death is £250 000. The official cost to the state is therefore £1 030 000 000. However, the EU figure for a statistical death is put at £1 000 000 – four times that to the UK – and the cost to the state therefore increases to £4 120 000 000. This represents about 8% of the public sector borrowing requirement.

# GENERAL PRACTICE CONSULTATIONS AND UNEMPLOYMENT

Dr Beale[12] was a GP in Calne, Wiltshire, at a time when the only factory in the town closed down. Examining his GP records, he found that, as soon as the threat of closure became known, consultations with those under threat of redundancy increased to 20% above previous attendance rates. Consultations stayed at that rate when unemployment struck, and rose further to 57% above normal among those who were unemployed for two or more years. The finding of a 20% increase in consultations for unemployed people is independently supported by the General Household Survey statistics.[13] Further independent support can be found in Figure 2.1, which plots regional unemployment rate against the number of prescription

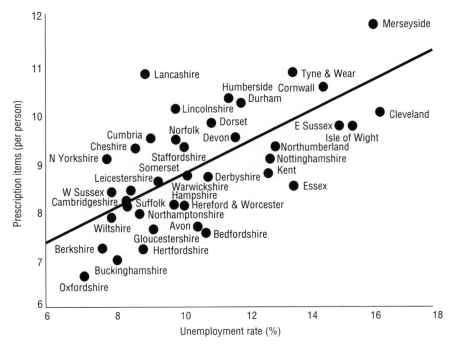

**Figure 2.1** Relationship between unemployment rate and prescription items per person by selected family health service authority (FHSA) 1993. Note that unemployment rates relate to December 1993 and are based on county data, the boundaries of which do not correspond to every one of the 90 FHSAs. As a result, only 39 out of 90 FHSAs are shown above. Source: PPA and Department of Employment.

items per person. It clearly shows that, the higher the unemployment rate is in a region, the higher the number of prescriptions that will be issued in that region.

Beale[12] also found that episodes of illness increased by 10.6% in those who were subject to the threat of loss of their jobs or unemployment itself. However, this was not a statistically significant increase.

One important aspect of this study in Calne is that at the time the town had a largely stable and closely knit population. Beale's findings therefore point to a relatively 'pure' effect of unemployment on health. Deprivation was not a problem for the two years when closure was threatened, although it would have entered the picture when unemployment began to bite. Possibly poverty was a factor in the further increase in consultation rates that was seen in the long-term unemployed.

The connection between unemployment and demand on health services is now so secure that Professor Mike Pringle[14] from the Department of General Practice at Nottingham University has argued that unemployment figures should be used for assessing the health needs of a locality. His team found that, in northern areas, both unemployment and prescribing costs were higher than in the south.

## The cost to the NHS of unemployment

One study[15] has estimated the extra cost to the NHS caused by unemployment as £71 million – £40.14 million in extra GP consultations and prescriptions and £30.6 million in lost prescription charges. This amounts to a 0.85% increase in the costs for primary care.

This estimate assumed a 20% increase in consultations for unemployed persons. The basis for this assumption is research carried out in Calne, quoted on page 13, and uses official government figures for unemployment.

The calculation can be reworked using UU index figures, which measure unemployment on a basis consistent with that officially in use before November 1982. Since that time 30 readjustments have been made to the way in which unemployment is counted, all of which have had the effect of reducing the figure.

According to the UU index, the number in unemployment in Autumn 1993 was 3 958 000. The average person consults his or her GP five times a year. If an unemployed person consults six times a year (a 20% increase), the additional burden of consultations caused by unemployment is one per unemployed person, i.e. an extra 3 958 000 consultations every year. The average cost of each GP consultation is £9.43, therefore the total cost of these additional consultations is 3 958 000 × £9.43 = £37 323 940 annually.

Seventy-two per cent of all GP consultations result in the issue of a prescription, thus unemployment results in an additional 3 958 000 × 72 = 2 849 760 prescriptions each year.

On average, only 87% of prescriptions are actually dispensed at the chemist; prescription charges deter some people. However, unemployed people do not pay these charges, so let us assume that 95% of their prescriptions, i.e. 2 849 760 × 95% = 2 707 272, are dispensed. The average prescription in 1993 cost £7.90, so the pharmaceutical bill that could be attributed to unemployment in 1993 was £21 387 449.

Unemployed people and their spouses pay no prescription charges to the NHS. This will add another £40 000 000 for the person and £4 000 000 for the spouse, assuming that one in ten is married.

The families of unemployed people also consult more. Let us take Beale's figures, who found that each employee had 1.3 dependants on average. This adds to the consultation bill: £37 323 940 × 1.3 = £48 521 122. And to the pharmaceutical bill for the families: £21 387 449 × 1.3 = £27 803 685.

The threat of redundancy causes people to consult more. Central Statistical Office figures[16] show that the redundancy rate by occupation was 11.9 – say ten per 1000 workers. The total workforce in 1993 was 20 882 000, so that 208 820 people were affected by redundancy. If the anxiety caused by the threat of redundancy affects this group for one year, it will cause 208 820 extra GP consultations.

The average cost of each GP consultation is £9.43; therefore the total cost for redundancy is 208 820 × £9.43 = £1 969 173.

Seventy-two per cent of all GP consultations result in the issue of a prescription so redundancy causes 208 820 × 72% = 150 350 prescriptions.

On average, only 87% of prescriptions are actually dispensed at the chemist so an extra 150 350 × 87% = 130 805 are dispensed as a result of redundancy.

The average prescription in 1992 cost £7.90, so the total pharmaceutical bill for redundancy was £1 033 360.

This gives a grand cost to family practitioner services of £172 728 727. The gross cost of family health services in 1990 was £6 800 000 000, so unemployment absorbs 2.5% of the total GP budget. It is a conservative figure, since it ignores the fact that the long-term unemployed consult 57% more.

An unquantifiable cost is the inefficiency created by the increased pressure on GPs' surgeries. Waiting times to see the GP will lengthen, with the resultant risk that some conditions may get worse. This effect can be moderated a little by the consideration that some other mild conditions may actually get better in the waiting time. The factor that remains is the extra stress on the primary health care services. Low morale leads to inefficiency and patient dissatisfaction, which leads, especially since the introduction of the new contract, to complaints, which completes a vicious circle by lowering morale still further.

A survey published in the *BMJ*[17] showed that one in four GPs shows signs of depression, nearly one-third has clinical levels of anxiety and some are so stressed that their decisions could be affected.

Beale[12] also found that hospital outpatient attendances were increased by 73% for those whose jobs were threatened or lost, and by 56% for their families. Taking 4 000 000 as the unemployment figure, and given that there is on average one outpatient attendance per year per head of population, this gives an extra 2 880 000 outpatient attendances. Each of these costs £48 at 1994–95 prices, which gives an extra cost of £138 240 000.

Assuming that each unemployed person has 1.3 dependants, (5 200 000 persons) and that they have an increased attendance rate of 56%, we have 2 912 000 extra outpatient attendances, at a cost of £139 776 000 to the NHS.

The cost of hospital inpatient treatment for diseases caused by unemployment cannot be ascertained.

In summary, a conservative and incomplete costing of the impact on NHS spending of treating illnesses attributable to unemployment is in the region of £1 116 506 373 (£1.1 billion) or 3.2% of the total budget. Since the increased demand on the NHS has not been budgeted for, this must be seen as a cut in NHS allocation. If this kind of cut were to be made overtly to the NHS budget, it would cause an outcry: it would simply be seen as politically unacceptable. The same reduction occurring indirectly as a result of external conditions has passed unnoticed.

# SMOKING AND ALCOHOL

The following workers have all come to the conclusion that unemployed people smoke more: Bradshaw *et al.*;[18] Cook *et al.*;[19] Warr and Payne;[20] Westcott;[21] and seven others. This may explain the high incidence of ischaemic heart disease (IHD, heart attacks and angina) that is seen in the unemployed, but is not likely to be the immediate cause of the higher incidence of lung cancer that was observed by Moser and Goldblatt,[1] since lung cancer takes many years to develop. A possible explanation for their observation is that the stress caused by unemployment may depress the immune reaction which had previously held the lung cancer in check.

Many cross-sectional studies have shown that unemployed men consume more cigarettes and alcohol than employed men.

The question of causality arises: does the stress of unemployment cause the increased rate or are heavy consumers more likely to lose their jobs?

Morris, Cook and Shaper[22] surveyed 6057 men, recording their weight, their self-assessment of smoking and drinking and their assessment of physical exercise. The study was limited by the fact that the period of time out of work was not assessed. They confirmed the previous findings that the unemployed smoked and drank more than those in work. However, they did not find that men increased their smoking or drinking on becoming unemployed; indeed, those who became non-employed through illness reduced their intake of both, probably in response to their doctors' advice. Unemployed men were more likely to reduce their alcohol intake, probably because they could not afford to go to the pub so often. They found that heavy smokers were more likely to lose their jobs. Although the stress and boredom of unemployment might be expected to drive people to drink and to smoke, it seems that this is offset by the financial hardship that it causes.

Other work on alcohol and unemployment contradicts the above findings. A total of 1083 pupils in a Swedish industrial town were interviewed during their last year of school, and then after two and five years.[23] They completed a questionnaire covering employment, alcohol consumption, education, migration and social background. Janlert and Hammerstrom[23] found that unemployed men and women drank twice as much alcohol as those who were in work, and that men moved from low intake to high intake on becoming unemployed. Factors contributing to high drinking patterns were stress and the amount of time available in which to drink. Income (or lack of it) did not appear to be a factor, despite the high cost of alcohol in Sweden. This contradicts evidence from other studies in which the amount consumed has been found to be proportional to the amount that the drinker can afford.

The conclusion is that the case for unemployment causing increased alcohol consumption is still 'unproven'.

# Weight gain, physical activity and serum cholesterol

Morris[22] found that 7.5% of the unemployed men reported that they had gained 10% more body weight as compared with only 5% of those who were employed. They were also more likely to be physically inactive. It is also reported that unemployment is associated with changes in blood cholesterol:[24] cholesterol concentrations rose when men became unemployed, and dropped when they found jobs.

## Heart attacks

If unemployed men have higher cholesterol levels, gain more weight, and smoke more; they are likely to suffer more heart attacks. A regional heart study[19] showed that the unemployed were more likely to suffer from IHD (any condition in which the blood supply to the heart is inadequate; the term covers both angina pectoris and heart attacks). However, because of the limitations of the study, it is not possible to conclude that the heart disease was caused by the job loss. It is surprising that there is not more research into this problem, since heart disease is one of the key areas for the Health of the Nation scheme.

# Mental health

There is a clear association between being unemployed and suffering from various mental symptoms. Clearly, a person whose mental health is not good is more likely to lose his or her job, but there is also good evidence that unemployment causes psychological misery. Three surveys show that about a fifth of the unemployed report that their mental health has deteriorated since losing their work, and the longer they remain out of work, the more likely they are to report deterioration. The symptoms reported are anxiety, worry, depression, unhappiness, dissatisfaction, neurosis, lower confidence, lower self-esteem and difficulty in sleeping.[25] An Australian study[26] of 16- to 24-year-olds showed that about half of unemployed people might be seen by a psychiatrist as worthy of treatment and, of a sample of 72, 28% had symptoms that came on after the onset of unemployment.

Clear evidence of the impact of unemployment on mental health was produced by Banks and Jackson,[27] who gave a general health questionnaire to 1000 16-year-old children in Leeds before and after they left school. Those who found work remained healthy, but those who did not showed evidence of deterioration in mental health. Importantly, there was no significant difference in the groups at the point at which they left school. Moreover, when they found jobs, their measured psychological health returned to normal levels. This evidence is all the more persuasive as young people are not so upset by unemployment as are older people, possibly because they may treat their leisure as a prolonged school holiday.

## The cost of mental stress

If we take it that four million people are unemployed, and that half of these are in need of treatment, but that only half of this group actually receive help, we are looking at one million people who need psychiatric treatment as a result of unemployment.

A very rough estimate of the annual cost of this treatment is the cost of one million people being seen once a month in a psychiatric outpatient department at £40 per consultation, i.e. one million × 12 × 40 = £480 000 000.

To estimate the drug costs, let us assume that 80% of people who are seen are treated with a cheap and standard antidepressant, Prothiaden tablets 75 mg, which cost £3.50 per month, while the remaining 20% are treated with a newer serotonin synaptic reuptake inhibitor (SSRI) antidepressant, Prozac, which costs £20.77 per month, and that each patient receives a six-month course of treatment. For Prothiaden the costs are 800 000 × £3.50 × 6 = £16 800 000. For Prozac the costs are 200 000 × £20.77 × 6 = £24 924 000. An incomplete estimate of the total annual cost to the NHS for mental illness caused by unemployment therefore comes to approximately £522 000 000.

If tranquillizers are prescribed for an anxiety/stress component, the costs are likely to be very much higher, because if they are taken for more than two weeks there is a high probability of dependence developing, which leads to a lifetime of drug taking. The January 1995 cost for 100 Valium 5 mg tablets was £2.81. A 40-year-old put on Valium for three weeks who becomes addicted and takes three per day until his death at 60 will run up a drugs bill of £61 370. The number of people for whom Valium and the like is being newly prescribed is available on the VAMP database, which contains full current prescribing habits of 500 GPs in the UK and which was donated to the government by Reuters. Unfortunately, the charge for obtaining the data is beyond the means of an individual researcher and therefore this information cannot be included here.

## Suicide and attempted suicide

In 1990 there were 5946 cases of suicide, self-inflicted injury and undetermined injuries in England and Wales. This rate is the second lowest in Europe after Greece. The incidence of suicide peaked in the 1930s at the time of the Depression when unemployment was high, and peaked again in the late 1950s and early 1960s, when unemployment was not a major problem. Over the last ten years in the UK, the incidence of young male suicides has risen by 71%.

Established factors that are linked with suicide are: boarding house accommodation, immigration, divorce, drug dependence, personality disorder, schizophrenia, epilepsy and chronic (i.e. long-lasting) pain and student life. Marital state has an effect on suicide rates. High rates are found among the divorced, and the rates become progressively lower for widow/ers, those never married, with the lowest rates among those who are married. Wives will be interested to note that suicide rates indicate that husbands are more content with their lot than their spouses, which probably reflects the dominant position assumed by males within marriage.

There is evidence that suicides are more common in social classes I and V at the extremes of the social spectrum. The availability of the means of suicide is a significant factor in the incidence of suicide.

Several researchers have found a positive relationship between suicide and unemployment.[28–32]

Pritchard's[30] work compared the rise in suicide rates in European Union (EU) countries from 1972 to 1988 with the rise in unemployment over the same period. The conclusions of the paper are as follows.

1   In the UK and in most other EU countries, youth suicide rates rose more than the general rates.
2   The youth suicide rate in the UK increased more than that in most other EU countries.
3   There were statistically significant associations between unemployment and general and youth suicide in the UK and most other EU countries, although the link was weaker in respect of youth suicide rates.

In an important official review of statistics[33] McColl quotes Bulusu and Alderson[34] as showing a negative relationship between unemployment and suicide. This is based on their remark that 'over the complete period there is no symmetry in the peaks and troughs of the numbers of suicides at all ages of males and the curve of unemployment'. However, in the next sentence they go on to say that 'Comparison with Figure 3 shows the greatest similarity with the trend for suicides in males aged 22–44', that is the age group most likely to be adversely affected by unemployment. Superimposition of the two graphs does indeed show a similarity in peaks and troughs for the two trends. The notable difference lies in the downward trend in suicide in the mid-1960s that resulted from the removal of poisonous carbon monoxide from the gas supplies.

Further, in a table setting out suicides by economic position, the standardized mortality ratio for economically inactive males is 184, and that for single females is 385. These are probably significant increases in the rates that would normally be expected ('probably' because statistical calculations to show the degree of certainty are not presented in the tables).

Another paper which was quoted by Population Health Outcome Indicators for the NHS as reporting a negative relationship between suicide and unemployment was that of Crombie,[35] who looked at unemployment rates in Scotland as a whole and at its constituent regions, and compared them with suicide rates. In fact, both conditions show a steep increase between 1979 and 1982. Statistically, there was one chance in a hundred that the similarity may have been due to coincidence, so this is not seen as a statistically significant increase – only one in a thousand or more is considered to be significant. There was no similarity for the rates for women, who might be less adversely affected by being out of a job.

In comparing regional unemployment and suicide rates, Crombie[35] found that the group of districts with low unemployment in 1971 but which experienced a large increase in unemployment to 1981 had overall the largest increase in suicide, but that the increase was not statistically significant. Crombie recognized that his negative or weakly positive findings contrasted with the findings from other workers, and reasoned that 'the impact of unemployment may depend on chances of re-employment and on local attitudes to employment state...some types of unemployment, such as the closure of a local steel works or coal mine, may have a different impact from others'.

Crombie's final conclusion was, 'I have found an association between trends in unemployment and suicide rates among men nationally but not regionally. These data do not support a rise in unemployment being a direct cause of the recent large increase in suicide among men.' These two sentences sit somewhat oddly together. Epidemiological studies can never, by their nature, give direct evidence of causality. It would not be correct, however, to say that Crombie found a negative association between suicide and unemployment.

Both of the papers quoted in authoritative official documents as refuting a connection between suicide and unemployment in fact contain material that supports the connection. It is surprising that official statistical work should make such elementary errors of data interpretation.

Suicide is a Health of the Nation key area. One of the best means of achieving the target of 15% reduction from the 1990 rate by the year 2000 will be to tackle the problem of unemployment directly.

Parasuicide (attempted suicide) shows a strong relationship with unemployment. For every employed person who makes a suicide attempt, there are 11 unemployed people who carry out the same act. For those out of work for more than one year, this figure rises to 19.[36,37] This is clear evidence of the human misery caused by unemployment.

No central statistics are kept for parasuicide. Estimates have been made by extrapolating from local figures; 87 000 admissions (D Gunnell, personal communication) or 120 000 attendances per year in England and Wales.[38] Given that 11 out of 12 are associated with unemployment, let us assume that only 50% are actually caused by unemployment. For 60 000 cases, this is the invoice:

*The bill for attempted suicide due to unemployment*

| | |
|---|---:|
| GP call out: assume 1:10 is a night visit @ £40: | £240 000 |
| GP visit, out of hours for 5:10 @ £15 | £450 000 |
| Ambulance for 50% of cases @ £50 | £3 000 000 |

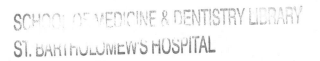

| | |
|---|---|
| Accident and emergency treatment for 120 000 @ £27 each | £3 240 000 |
| Two days in hospital bed for 43 500 @ £286 each | £12 441 000 |
| Psychiatrist visit in hospital for 40 000 @ £20 | £800 000 |
| Psychiatric follow-up: assume two outpatient visits @ £40 for 20 000 | £1 600 000 |
| Total cost to NHS of parasuicide due to unemployment: | £21 771 000 |

The cost of unemployment-associated suicide can be assessed from population risk and the imputed cost of death.

Fox[39] found that the unemployed were two to three times more likely to commit suicide than average, and Moser found the risk to be doubled.

Given that the death rate for suicide and undetermined injury is ten per 100 000 of the general population, the unemployed population will have an extra ten per 100 000, or 400 for an unemployed population of four million. If we assume that each suicide costs the state £1 000 000, the cost to the state of this problem is therefore £400 million per year. This will not be counted separately as it will be included in the bill for total mortality.

## Health of the Nation

Three of these effects (smoking, heart attacks and suicide) are Health of the Nation key areas, that is problems which are targeted for special attention. There is therefore very good reason for the government to target unemployment as a priority problem to be tackled if it wished to achieve the targets set.

In conclusion, there is no reasonable doubt that unemployment is associated with an increase in suicide and parasuicide rates. This fact further strengthens the evidence that unemployment causes mental ill-health, since suicide and attempted suicide do not occur out of the blue: they are merely the measurable tip of an iceberg of misery.

Since unemployment causes psychological ill-health, it follows that at least part of the observed physical ill-health is also caused by rather than merely associated with unemployment, since we know that mind and body are part of a whole and that mental stress will necessarily result in physical illness.

## THE IMPACT OF UNEMPLOYMENT ON THE PERSON

Psychological studies have been carried out on unemployed individuals. Using separate approaches, Jahoda[40] and Warr[41] have come to similar conclusions, namely that work is an important and beneficial factor in the well-being of an individual.

Their separate findings can be fused to form the following conclusions.

1   *Work gives structure to time and activity.* It gives a pattern to the day, preventing time from being a series of intervals between rising, eating, smoking and going to bed.

2   *Work gives status.* This is not merely derived from the financial rewards of working and the freedom of choice offered by possession of money, but people taking satisfaction from using skills that they already possess, and in acquiring new skills. A working person gains a sense of self-respect.

3   *Work gives social contact and social stimulation.* One is unlikely to be lonely in a workplace; and in addition to this sense of company, there is another benefit of cooperating with others in realizing social goals, which go beyond narrow individual aims.

4   *Work gives a sense of security*; both financial and social, to working people and their families.

These are all powerful, creative psychological determinants. The negative impact of unemployment on mental health has been confirmed by Dr Philip Taylor of the Department of Sociological Studies at Sheffield University in a detailed review of the scientific literature.[42]

Tabloid journalists and right-wing politicians commonly characterize the unemployed as lazy, feckless people living a life of luxury at the expense of the taxpayer. This can only be seen as a form of scapegoating, a projection on to an outsider of attributes that the accusers do not wish to own up to in themselves. This kind of comment can only add to the distress already felt by the unemployed. Freedom of speech means that these opinions will continue to be expressed, so, as with most of the other problems associated with unemployment, the only answer seems to be to attack the problem at its root by enabling all those who wish to work to do so.

## UNEMPLOYMENT, DRUGS AND CRIME

'Old-fashioned commonsense' leads us to expect that unemployment would lead to an increase in crime: 'The Devil finds work for idle hands to do'. With time on their hands, living in a society where every street corner advertisement hoarding, newspaper, magazine and 50% of television stations urge us to desire consumer goods, it would be odd if some unemployed did not take to theft as a way of redressing the perceived imbalance in their lives.

Figure 2.2 shows the relationship between the unemployment rate and car crime on a regional basis. Clearly, the higher the unemployment rate, the more car crime is to be expected. The relationship for theft derived from the Regional Trends figures (Figure 2.3) is not so clear, although there is a suggestion of proportionality. It is tempting to speculate from these figures that simple, unskilled theft from cars (and joyriding) is the response of some individuals to the poverty caused by unemployment, but that more complex, daring and skilled theft such as burglary is not so strongly a simple response to unemployment. It might be that a spell in jail to learn the skills of burglary is necessary before the unemployed can take to housebreaking.

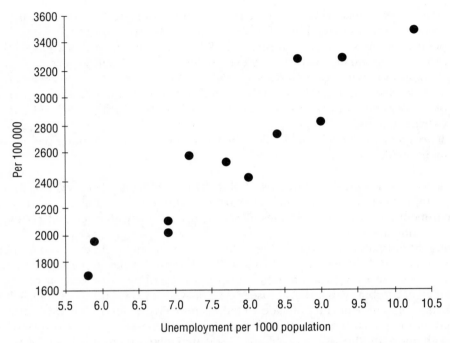

**Figure 2.2** Unemployment versus vehicle-related theft, by region, 1991. Source: Regional Trends.

These findings are being confirmed by senior police officers, who are beginning to voice what is to them common knowledge that petty theft and car crime in a given area are expected to rise in parallel with unemployment.

In contrast, the same regional data show no relationship between unemployment and vandalism (Figure 2.4).

The link between unemployment and crime is backed by Figure 2.5, which relates unemployment to crime over the years, and shows a parallel relationship between fluctuations of both. The graph is drawn from a study by John Wells of Cambridge University for the Employment Policy Institute, who concluded that there is a positive link between crime and both poverty and unemployment.

In view of this, it is surprising that sociologists in the past were unable to find any strong link between unemployment *per se* and crime.[43] It may be that the essence of the problem lies in the '*per se*'. Unemployment causes deprivation, and it is often impossible to separate the effects of unemployment and deprivation. This distinction is of more academic significance than practical.

Part of the explanation for this may be that it would be politically controversial to link unemployment with crime on two counts. At the time of writing, the Conservative Party is in Government, and accepts unemployment as a 'price worth paying'[44] to contain inflation. It would not wish that link to be made, especially as

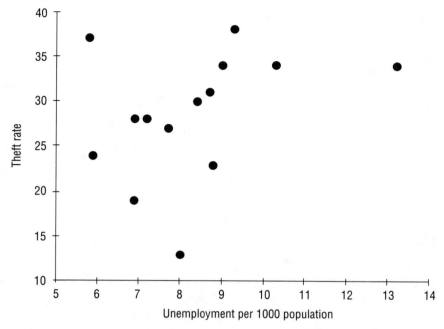

**Figure 2.3** Unemployment versus theft rates, by region, 1991. Source: Regional Trends.

it wishes to be seen as the party of 'law and order'. Opposition politicians, on the other hand, do not wish to be perceived to accuse the unemployed in general of being lawless. However, some right-wing politicians and many tabloid journalists are not above insinuating that the unemployed generally are idle, feckless, scroungers. In reality, the fact that a subsection of the unemployed turn to crime has no more implication for the majority than the fact that some MPs take money for asking questions.

The other argument that is commonly used in this debate is that the severe unemployment of the Great Depression of the 1930s did not cause a rise in crime. *Autres temps, autres moeurs.* The population of the 1930s lived in a different setting of social cohesion and morality. Social hierarchy and religion were stronger, or at least not so weak, and advertising and commercialism did not have the powerful hold on the national psyche that it now has. The experience of the 1930s has little direct relevance to the present situation.

Most importantly of all, illicit drug taking (apart from alcohol) was not part of the 1930s social scene. There is good evidence to link unemployment and illicit drugs, and hard drug addiction is most certainly linked with crime.

Cross-sectional studies have shown that drug abuse is associated with un-employment. The British Crime Survey of 1981 showed that cannabis use was

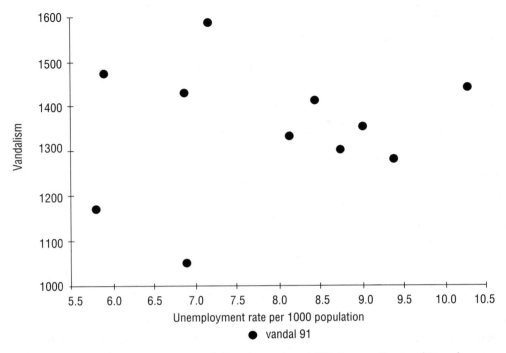

**Figure 2.4**  Unemployment versus vandalism, by region, 1991. Source: Regional Trends.

higher among the unemployed,[45] and unemployment was shown to be one of the characteristics of the subgroup most at risk of exposure to drugs.[46]

In a longitudinal study of almost a thousand Lothian teenagers, it was found that illicit drug use was significantly higher among those who were unemployed. The researchers found no evidence that those who later became unemployed were more drug orientated when at school. They also found that the longer a person was unemployed, the more likely he or she was to take drugs.[47,48]

In the Lothian study, it was found that, on average, employed men had been exposed to 0.5 illicit drugs. For the unemployed who were seeking work this figure was 1.4; but for those unemployed who had given up seeking work the figure was 2.8.

Given that cannabis is illegal, those seeking to buy cannabis are more likely to come into contact with dangerous drugs such as crack and heroin. The law drives the two together.

The conclusion is that there is evidence that unemployment causes an increase in crime through the relative deprivation that it causes and through the stimulus it gives to drug dependence.

In chapter 3 we shall look at the options for reducing the burden of unemployment on the NHS and the country as a whole.

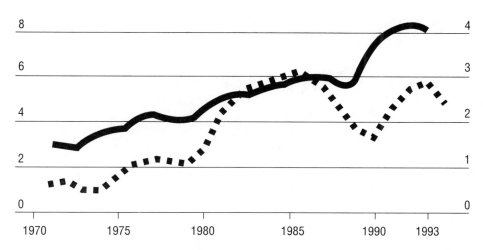

**Figure 2.5** Crime wave. *Solid line*: all property crime, England and Wales. Offences per 100 000 population, 000s, left-hand scale. *Dotted line*: annual average UK unemployment, millions, right-hand scale. Source: DoE, EPI.

# REFERENCES

1   Moser K A and Goldblatt P O (1986) Unemployment and mortality: further evidence from the OPCS longitudinal study 1971–91. *Lancet*: **i**; 365–6.

2   Townsend P, Phillimore P, Beattie A (1986) *Inequalities in Health in the Northern Region*. Northern Regional Health Authority and the University of Bristol, Bristol.

3   Brenner H (1979) *Mental illness and the economy*. Harvard University Press, Cambridge, Massachusetts.

4   Brenner H (1979) Mortality and the national economy: a review and the experience of England and Wales. *Lancet*: **2**; 568–73.

5   Brenner H (1980) Industrialisation and economic growth: estimates of their effects on the health of the population. In: H Brenner, A Mooney, T J Nagy (eds) *Assessing the contributions of the social sciences to health*. American Academy for the Advancement of Science.

6   Brenner H (1980) Importance of the economy to the nation's health. In: L Eisenberg and A Kleinman (eds) *The relevance of social science for medicine*. Reidel, New York.

7   Brenner H (1983) Mortality and economic instability: detailed analyses for Britain and comparative analyses for selected industrialised countries. *Int J Health Ser*: **13**; 563–620.

8   Gravelle H S E, Hutchinson G, Stern J (1981) Mortality and unemployment: a critique of Brenner's time series analysis. *Lancet*: **ii**; 675–9.

9   Moser K A, Fox A J, Jones D R (1984) Unemployment and mortality in the OPCS longitudinal study. *Lancet*: **ii**; 1324–9.

10  Gravelle H S E (1985) *Does unemployment kill?* York Portfolios, Nuffield, p. 9.

11  Scott-Samuel A (1984) Unemployment and Health. *Lancet*: **ii**; 1464–5.

12  Beale N R and Nethercott S (1986) Job loss and morbidity in a group of employees nearing retirement age. *J R Coll Gen Pract*: **36**; 265–6.

13  *General Household Survey* (1989 and 1990) Office of Population Censuses and Surveys, London.

14  Pringle M and Morton-Jones T (1994) Using unemployment rates to predict prescribing trends in England. *BJGP*: **44**; 53–6.

15  Griffin J (1993) *The Impact of Unemployment on Health*. Office of Health Economics, London.

16  Government Statistical Service (1995) *Labour, Market Data, Nov. 1994–Jan. 1995*, London.

17  Caplan R (1994) Stress, anxiety and depression in hospital consultants, general practitioners and senior health service managers. *BMJ*: **309**; 1261–3.

18  Bradshaw J, Cooke K, Godfrey C (1983) The impact of unemployment on the living standards of families. *J Soc Pol*: **12**; 433–52.

19  Cook D G, Cummins R O, Bartly M J *et al*. (1982) Health of unemployed middle aged men in Great Britain. *Lancet*: **i**; 1290–4.

20  Warr P and Payne R (1983) Social class and reported changes in behaviour after job loss. *J Appl Soc Psych*: **13**; 206–22.

21  Westcott G (1985) The effect of unemployment on the health of workers in a UK steel town. In: G Westcott, P G Svensson and H F K Zollner (eds) *Health policy implications of unemployment*. World Health Organization, Copenhagen.

22  Morris J K, Cook D G, Shaper A G (1992) Non-employment and changes in smoking, drinking and bodyweight. *BMJ*: **304**; 536–41.

23  Janlert O and Hammerstrom A (1992) Alcohol consumption among unemployed youths: results from a prospective study. *Br J Addict*: **87**; 703–14.

24  Jahoda M (1979) The impact of unemployment in the 1930s and the 1970s. *Bull Br Psychol Soc*: **32**; 309–14.

25  Warr P (1985) Twelve questions about unemployment and health. In: R Roberts, R Finnegan, D Gallie (eds) *New Approaches to Economic Life*. Manchester University Press, Manchester.

26  Finlay-Jones R and Eckhardt B (1981) Psychiatric disorder among the young unemployed. *Aus NZ J Psychiat*: **15**; 265–70.

27  Banks M H and Jackson P R (1982) Unemployment and risk of minor psychiatric disorder in young people: cross sectional and longitudinal evidence. *Psychol Med*: **12**; 897–8.

28    Swinscow D (1951) Some suicide statistics. *BMJ*. **1**; 1417–22.

29    Sainsbury P (1955) *Suicide in London*. Chapman & Hall, London.

30    Pritchard C (1992) Is there a link between suicide in young men and unemployment? *Br J Psychiat*. **160**; 750–6.

31    Diekstra R W F (1989) Suicide and attempted suicide: an international perspective. *Acta Psychiat Scand*. **80**; 1–24.

32    Dooley D, Catalano R, Rook K *et al.* (1989) Economic stress and suicide: multi-variate analysis of economic stress and suicidal ideation. Part 2. *Suicide Life Threat Behav*. **19**; 337–51.

33    McColl A J and Gulliford M C (1993) *Population Health Outcome Indicators for the NHS. A feasibility study*. Faculty of Public Health Medicine, London.

34    Bulusu L and Alderson M (1984) Suicides 1950–82. *Popul Trends*. **35**; 11–17.

35    Crombie I K (1986) Trends in suicide and unemployment in Scotland between 1976 and 1986. *BMJ*. **298**; 782–4.

36    Platt S (1984) Unemployment and suicidal behaviour. *Soc Sci Med*. **19**; 93–115.

37    Hawton K and Rosse N (1986) Unemploymment and attempted suicide among men in Oxford. *Health Trends*. **18**; 29–32.

38    Hawton K and Fagg J (1992) Trends in deliberate self poisoning and self injury in Oxford 1976–90. *BMJ*. **304**; 1409–11.

39    Fox A J and Shewry (1988) New longitudinal insights into relationships between unemployment and mortality. *Stress Med*. **4**; 11–19.

40    Jahoda M (1979) The impact of unemployment in the 1930s and the 1970s. *Bull Br Psychol Soc*. **32**; 309–14.

41    Warr P B (1991) *Work, unemployment and mental health*. Oxford Science Publications, Oxford.

42    Taylor P (1991) *Unemployment and health. Campaign for work research report, Vol. 3, No. 6*. Campaign for work, Annexe B, Tottenham Town Hall, London.

43    Horowitz A V (1984) The economy and social pathology. *Ann Rev Sociol*. **10**; 95–119.

44    Norman Lamont (1991) House of Commons, London.

45    Mott H J (1981) Self reported cannabis use in Great Britain in 1981. *Br J Addict*. **80**; 34–73.

46    Research International (1986) *Heroin misuse evaluation campaign*. Research Bureau, London.

47    Plant M A, Peck D F, Samuel D (1986) *Alcohol, drugs and school leavers*. Tavistock, London.

48    Peck D F and Plant M A (1986) Unemployment and illegal drug use: concordant evidence from a prospective study and national trends. *BMJ*. **293**; 929–32.

# 3

# Solutions to the problem of unemployment

## DO NOT ADJUST REALITY, THERE IS A FAULT WITH YOUR ECONOMICS

Work is a necessary part of biological existence. Even the amoeba does work in the act of moving towards and engulfing its food. Aboriginal peoples living in a state of harmony and balance with their surroundings nevertheless have to work in hunting, gathering and shelter building, although it is humbling for us to consider that they spend far less of their time 'at work' and far more of their time simply resting, talking and celebrating together than we who are surrounded by the 'labour-saving' trappings of our 'civilization'.[1]

Work can be considered as a way of lessening the entropy (that is increasing the order) in our personal environment. As any parent of a two-year-old child knows, there is a natural tendency for the environment to move towards a state of chaos, where everything is randomly intermingled. Much of the work of parenthood is reducing this state of disorder, separating, and teaching separation of, food from playthings, playthings from life-threatening objects such as fire and roadways, and so on. Life-sustaining, non-alienated work (as opposed to indirect forms of work or 'employment' in which the immediate aim is to earn money) requires selecting from the environment the resources required to satisfy our need for food, water, shelter and warmth.[2]

There is also a necessity to avoid contaminating our food, water and immediate environment with our own biological waste products, that is to order the place where we excrete.

All too often, economists lose sight of the biological foundation of our lives so that the ecological system on which the human economy ultimately depends is

classed as a 'market externality', which is a cost-free 'datum' (literally, given).
Realization of the error of this old thinking is percolating slowly into the consciousness of the average economist, and new economic thinking is emerging that
seeks to bring ecological realities into the economic realm.[3] 'Sustainable development' is nominally accepted as the new paradigm of economic thinking, a phrase
which adorns many treaties and papers, but whose true meaning is lost on the
majority of political leaders.

Sustainable development was introduced in the Brundtland Report,[4] and defined
as development that satisfies the needs of the present generation without compromising the ability of future generations to meet their needs. Although touted as a
moderate definition, and set against the perceived excesses of those who call for a
steady-state economy, consideration of the projected explosion of the human
population suggests that to apply this literally would mean a very considerable
contraction in our own standard of living.

Alternative definitions of sustainable development include the remarkable effort
of Pearce,[5] who offers: 'continuously rising, or at least non-declining consumption
per capita, or GNP, or whatever the agreed indicator of development is'.

This suggests that there is open season on definitions, and so the following is
offered:

> Sustainable development is human development in its widest sense – economic,
> social, scientific, technological, intellectual, cultural and spiritual – that maximizes
> equity in three ways:
>
> - between rich and poor in a nation
> - between rich and poor nations
> - between present and future generations.

While these debates proceed, back in the real world there is a vast amount of
good work crying out to be done in order to protect and stabilize the environment. It is simply illogical to have 10% or more of the potential workforce
excluded from employment while this work remains undone. If the prevailing
economic system is unable to make the connection between the twin imperatives
of environmental protection and job creation, then the system is faulty and must
be amended.

In fact, the fault comes not so much from economists as from a wilful misunder-
standing of the realities of the situation by key decision makers. Whenever environmental protection is mentioned, politicians and pundits alike reiterate the
mis-statement that it is necessary to have conventional economic growth in order
to create the wealth necessary to protect the environment. This disregards the fact
that it is conventional economic activity that is degrading the environment in the
first place. It is like the man who dragged a log around in order to have something
to sit on when he became tired. Like the 'trickle down' theory that wealth given to
the rich would improve the lot of the poor, which is also devoid of any basis in
objective reality, this statement still enjoys wide acceptance, and goes unchal-

lenged except on the rare occasions that an environmentalist is present in a political discussion. A discussion paper published by Friends of the Earth (FoE)[6] has dealt a body blow to this fallacy; as it is the source for many of the figures in this chapter, it will be referred to simply as FoE.

The premise of this chapter is therefore that both unemployment and environmental degradation are incompatible with the true meaning of sustainable development, but that these two problems may be merged to form a single solution.

## THE FINANCIAL COSTS OF UNEMPLOYMENT

We have seen in chapter 2 the human cost and the cost to the NHS imposed by unemployment. In following chapters we will also assess the costs of the poverty that follows from unemployment. Some people are contemptuous of bleeding-heart contemplations of human suffering, so another cost is set out here: the financial cost to the taxpayer of unemployment (Table 3.1).

- The total of £26 576 million amounts to over £9000 per unemployed person.
- Lost output would amount to between 5% and 8% of the gross domestic product.
- The cost to the state of social security benefits is multiplying: in 1992–93 it was £9 290 000 000 – three times larger than the figure for 1979–80.
- Piachaud[7] reasons that 'it is realistic to think of unemployment as imposing a tax equivalent of ten pence on basic rate income tax'.

The administration of the benefits system at the time of writing is a nightmare. Half of all households receive means-tested benefits, a system that is complex and facilitates cheating. It is well known that there is widespread bending of the rules. Sixty per cent of fraudulent claims come from undeclared earnings. Organized fraud accounts for 9% of the losses, at an estimated cost of £60 million per year.

**Table 3.1**   Costs of unemployment for 1994

|  | £ million |
|---|---|
| Benefits to unemployed | 10 816 |
| Extra disablement | 4 004 |
| Administration | 640 |
| Taxes foregone |  |
| Direct | 4 581 |
| National insurance contributions | 3 371 |
| Indirect taxes | 3 164 |
| Total | £26 576 |

Source: Piachaud,[7] Employment Policy Institute Paper 8.6.

Since unemployment causes sickness, and also causes people to claim Sickness Benefit since that is a larger pay cheque, we should look also at the Sickness Benefit budget. Piachaud[7] estimates that at least one-third of the growth in expenditure on the long-term sick and disabled is due to the growth in unemployment. This is deduced from the fact that, between 1979 and 1993, Sickness Benefit payments rose by 9.8% when unemployment was rising, but only by 5.5% when it was falling.

The costs for policing, criminal justice, social services and health have not been included in this equation, but these incomplete figures are surely enough to convince that society cannot reasonably bear the financial, let alone the human, costs of unemployment. It is clear that something must give. Only a fool would conclude that the answer is to reduce the Unemployment Benefit, further increasing poverty: but what other options are there?

# WHAT HOPE FOR REDUCING UNEMPLOYMENT?

## Workfare

Some politicians of the right respond to the problem of unemployment by arguing that the unemployed should go on to workfare – a benefit whose receipt depends on carrying out work assigned to the claimant. The unemployed are workshy, they argue, and are happy to sponge from those worthy souls who do work. They should be made to work for their benefit, and that would motivate them to go out and get a proper job. The extreme right-wing press gives much prominence to cases of benefit fraud, with the effect that most claimants are tainted with guilt by association.

History will look back and condemn a party that created unemployment in order to curb wages and increase international competitiveness, only to accuse the victims of this policy of being idle. It is perfectly clear that the vast majority of those who have lost their jobs have not chosen to leave work – they have been made redundant. It may well be that there is a new generation coming through for whom the concept of a regular job is unknown, and who have no work ethic, but this is again hardly their fault, but rather the result of increasing mechanization of work and the competitive necessity of reducing wage costs.

It is unconscionable therefore that people who have lost their jobs through no fault of their own should be stigmatized as 'spongers' and effectively punished with a loss of personal liberty to choose what form of work they will follow through the imposition of workfare. It is a short step from this scheme to the philosophy of the workhouse and the work camp. Forced labour is degrading for the worker and inefficient for the system that employs it. It is a truism in the Forces that one volunteer is worth ten conscripts. Anger and resentment created by workfare could act as the spark that sets off widespread social unrest.

Apologists for workfare may ask why society should pay any benefit to someone who will not contribute. However, society is in fact already putting a condition on most benefits that debars the claimant from contributing through gainful employment. The key to progress is not to react emotionally with a return to forced labour, but to remove the condition that stops a claimant from working – the 'available for work' clause. Of which more later (see p. 40).

# Economic growth?

The orthodox prescription of ministers and frontbenchers of both parties for reducing unemployment is to create conditions favourable for economic growth. Growth will stimulate production, they believe, and jobs will follow. Unfortunately, it is not quite as simple as that, on four counts:

1  economic cycles
2  the disparity of growth and employment creation
3  the non-sustainability of indefinite economic growth
4  technological innovation where machines displace human workers.

## Economic cycles

For a variety of reasons, capitalized economies are prone to regular cycles of peaks and troughs of activity. During the troughs, jobs are shed as fast as a dog sheds hair in spring time. Governments seem powerless to prevent these troughs from happening, although they do seem to be capable of making them worse, as happened for instance with Nigel Lawson's boom of 1987, which intensified the subsequent recession. The recession itself was blamed with partial justification on the worldwide recession that was and is taking place. These cycles mean that jobs gained on the swings of growth will be lost again on the roundabouts of recessions.

## Disparity of growth and employment creation

One calculation[8] concluded that in order to create 3.5 million jobs over a five-year period at a rate of 700 000 per year, annual economic growth of 5.75% would be needed. The real trend in growth in the UK and for most other developed economies stands at 2.5%. High growth rates of 4–5% are possible when starting from a low base, but have never been sustained. Even if it were possible to attain 5% growth per year indefinitely, there would be enormous inflationary pressures in the economy, which would make the growth fail sooner or later – probably sooner. Investment aimed at increasing the productive capacity of the economy and available skills in the workforce to meet increasing demand could perhaps bring growth up to 3 or 4% for a period, but even this would inevitably come up against the limit of inflation.

## Unsustainability of conventional economic growth

In the real world, nothing can grow forever. A tree may grow for hundreds of years, but eventually will stop growing and die. A human being grows from birth to the age of 18 or so, and there growth stops. A population of any living species, without exception, can grow until its demands exceed one or more of three natural constraints:

1 the area of its habitat
2 supply of nutrients
3 negative feedback created by the toxins that it excretes.

These constraints certainly apply to the human population. They are incontrovertible biological truths with which no scientist or philosopher would disagree.

Orthodox political economists place their economic theories outside of these biological systems and claim that economic growth or development can continue indefinitely. There is a real philosophical problem here, since political economists are claiming as an article of faith that a biological system, namely the human population, which is engaged in consuming resources both irreplaceable (coal, oil, gas, uranium, minerals) and renewable (fish, forests and soil) can continue to grow indefinitely and without constraint. The only inference that can be made is that orthodox economics is not a science in the sense of a search for ideas that are congruent with a real world existing 'out there'. Rather it must be a closed belief system that is to some extent internally self-consistent, but which cannot bear any exposure to physical reality, rather like the belief system of the mediaeval scholastic who refused to look into Galileo's telescope for fear that what he might see there would contradict Aristotle.

Abraham Lincoln believed that it was impossible to fool all people all the time. He reckoned without the advent of modern means of communication. It is a real testimony to the ability of the modern political system, working in alliance with the instruments of mass information, that thinkers who challenge the doctrine of economic growth should be seen as in error, rather than those who propagate the impossible notion that indefinite growth is possible in a closed system.

It is true to say that over the period 1989 to 1995 the argument has progressed a little. The point at which the human economy actually affects the surrounding world is in its 'throughput' – that is, the amounts that it extracts from the world as minerals, for example, and the amount of pollution it causes as emissions of sewage and other wastes. It is true also that benign economic growth will be possible when we begin to act to diminish throughput by changing the economy from a linear footing (extract–manufacture–use–dispose) to a cyclical footing (manufacture, reuse, recycle). At this point in history we are in the happy position of being able to obtain benign growth ('green growth') through investing and creating activity in sectors such as pollution control.

Unfortunately, ministers are more at pains to reiterate the falsehood that environmental protection will be expensive than to create the conditions whereby industries are able to manufacture the hardware of environmental protection on a competitive basis.

We must recognize that perfection is not possible, so that even the most steady-state economy can only minimize throughput; it is not likely to be possible to eliminate it altogether. This consideration should not deter us from setting about reducing present emissions.

The conclusion is that, even if it were possible by economic growth alone to bring about full employment (which it is not), the reality is that economic growth would collapse in the long term. Economic growth alone, or coupled with investment and training, cannot bring back full employment.

## Technological innovation

The introduction of machines to do work previously carried out by humans is an intrinsic part of economic growth. Machines increase productivity and lower wage costs, but increase capital costs. Computerization is reputed to decrease human work, although anyone who has had anything to do with computerization of an office may choose to disagree. Robotics may certainly displace workers, and this effect may be welcomed in the sense that it frees workers from mind-numbing and dehumanizing work that effectively reduces them to the status of an extension of a machine. It is sometimes argued that computers will slavishly take all work from us, creating our wealth for us so that the entire human population can look forward to a life of indefinite luxury reminiscent of the upper classes of the Roman empire. Others restrict the outlook for computers to do routine tasks, and reserve work in the environment – housebuilding, farming, countryside management and the like – to humans, who are possibly better suited for this kind of work. Whatever the ultimate outcome, technological innovation puts the lid on any hope that economic growth will provide anything but a partial answer to the problem of unemployment.

# Training schemes

One of the weaknesses of the UK economy is that our manufacturing is of the 'pile-'em-high and sell-'em-cheap' variety. As such, it is competing against the newly industrialized 'tiger' economies where labour costs are a fraction of our own. In some parts of China, labour costs actually stand at zero, since the labour is slave labour of prisoners, some of whom may be political dissidents. In view of this it would be reasonable to institute tariffs and bans that reflect bad social and environmental practices implicit in some cheap imported goods. Unfortunately, the General Agreement on Tariffs and Trade (GATT) rules out this kind of action: our workers are expected to continue to compete against workers whose wages and conditions are set at a very much lower level.

One necessary response is to increase the skills of our workforce so that they are able to produce complex, high-technology products. Free market ideology dictates that this training should be provided by the private sector. Unfortunately, if a private sector employer invests in training a worker, there is no guarantee that the fully-trained worker may not leave when qualified, possibly to take up a position with a competitor who can afford to pay higher wages, precisely because they make savings on their training budget. Training for understanding of environmental protection measures is also needed.[9] For this reason, government investment in training would be wise and practical.

## Redistributing work – shorter working week and job sharing

In a recent survey it was found that 44% of the UK workforce returned from work exhausted, compared with only 17% in The Netherlands. Stress due to work may be costing 10% of GNP per year.

It is illogical that some members of the workforce should be stressed because they have no work, while a proportion of the remainder should be made stressed because they are working too hard. A report by the London School of Economics into the effects of the reduction of the working week from 39 to 37 hours showed that, under the shorter regimen, productivity rose and attitudes in the workforce became happier. Overtime did not rise, so the new hours increased employment at no extra cost.

Job sharing is a reasonable response to the fact that work itself is stressful and worklessness is also stressful. The drawbacks are twofold: first, people in work who share their jobs must be prepared to take a cut in income. This is often not as impossible as it seems. The gain in quality of life through decreased pressure is greater than the loss in quality from decreased income. Second, the two job sharers must be able to communicate efficiently with their job-sharing partners. This causes a degree of increased work for the partners, but it is not an insuperable problem. In the end, it is the attitude of employers to job sharing which is the determining factor, and doubtless as time goes on the idea will gradually become more acceptable.

## Training for leisure

The redistribution of work means increased leisure for all. Forward-thinking employers offer classes to prepare retiring colleagues for their leisure. Work imposes structure and rhythm to time, provides social contacts and gives a sense of purpose to life. Deliberate planning is needed to replace these structures and qualities to life outside of formal work. Educational facilities provided by the community free or at low cost to those facing long periods out of formal work would be a reasonable investment in the happiness of those involved. Redistribution of work and a positive view of increased leisure is helpful, but cannot be seen as the sole response to worklessness.

## Local exchange and trading systems (LETS)

Not all people react badly to unemployment. The loss of boring, low-paid and stress-ful work is not hard to bear. There is evidence also that a certain type of person who is active, is good at organizing time and has a sense of purpose, whether political, religious or personal, is protected against the harmful effects of unemployment.[10] Local exchange and trading systems are ideally suited to being set up by such people, who will be able to use the scheme to devote their talents and energies use-fully within their communities, drawing others along in the wake of their energy.

Local exchange and trading systems are essentially a more developed form of barter. In setting up such a scheme, a group of people with a range of skills to offer come together around a database. A computer is helpful but not essential. Each is allocated an equal number of credits, say 50, which can be called 'creds', with which they may trade within a LETS area. Alice may use her handyperson skills to fix Brian's shed door; she gains five creds, and Brian loses five, but regains them by babysitting for Cathy, and so on. The account of each and every member is available for inspection by all, so that members who consistently take more than they give will soon find that others lose interest in doing things for them until they have repaid creds to the pool.

These schemes are highly successful in stimulating meaningful local economic activity irrespective of the amount of cash that may or may not exist in the locality. Some LETS creds interface with formal currency, with some shops accepting payment in part or whole in creds. The Inland Revenue has formally inspected the way the scheme works and has decided not to get involved, so that LETS income need not be declared on tax forms, nor need it affect a person's entitlement to benefits.

Local exchange and trading systems are becoming increasingly common in North America and the Anglophone countries. At the end of 1994 there were approximately 300 schemes in the UK. It is a valuable auxiliary service to a defec-tive macroeconomy, but makes no claims to replace the need for a monetary economy. However, if the formal monetary economy at any stage should collapse under the weight of its own internal contradictions, it is possible that LETS will play a central part in the regeneration of a new, rational economy.[a]

## Tax reform

There is a growing awareness of the advantages that would accrue from shifting the burden of taxation away from 'goods' and on to 'bads'; away from jobs and on to consumption of material resources and other practices that need to be discour-aged on environmental grounds.[11] National insurance contributions and income

[a] For more information send six second-class stamps to LetsLink, 65 Woodcock Road, Warminster BA12 9DH, UK.

tax both increase the cost of labour (which now meets 50% of the tax burden in the EU), with the result that pressures increase on employers to shed jobs. A European Commission investigation[12] into the effects of a $10/barrel carbon tax on oil with an equivalent reduction in employers' social security contributions estimated that a total of 650 000 jobs would be created in six EU countries. Of these, 150 000 would be in the UK, of which 69 000 would be in industry and 43 000 in services. So much for the idea that environmental measures are not good for the economy. This was merely for a carbon tax: eco-taxes should also be applied to all finite resources, and to polluting practices of all kinds. Another virtue of resource taxes are that they are easy to apply and difficult to evade compared with income taxes: but a disadvantage is that they lack the progressive virtues of income tax – that is, they do not automatically fall harder on the rich. However, given the political will, it would be possible to structure taxes so that the rich pay more and the poor pay less so that the net effect is to produce convergence (increasing income equality) in the economy. One of the key factors in bringing this about would be the introduction of a citizen's income scheme (see below), which is strongly progressive in effect.

# Citizen's Income and wage subsidy

The citizen's income (CI) or basic income scheme proposes that a benefit is paid unconditionally and universally to all citizens of a country. Its level will vary with age, and those with special needs may receive supplementary benefits, but otherwise it is paid to all, regardless of whether or not they work, and regardless of their level of income. It is aimed at meeting the costs of basic subsistence, and can be seen as the modern equivalent of the right of a pastoralist to own a piece of land on which to earn a livelihood.

The great advantage of a CI is that it breaks people out of the traps of unemployment and poverty.

## Breaking the traps

Unemployment Benefit, which is soon to be replaced by the Job Seekers' Allowance, and Income Support both come on condition that the recipient must be available for, and indeed actively seeking, employment. A small 'earnings disregard' allows those receiving Unemployment Benefit to earn up to £2 per day (£12 per week), and a similar amount of added earnings is possible on Income Support, but any more than that leads to loss of benefit. Recipients may do no more that 16 hours of unpaid voluntary work per week. The effect is that claimants receive the dole on condition that they do no work. If they do find work, their benefit is effectively subject to 100% marginal taxation, so that for many people, especially unskilled low-wage earners in receipt of Housing Benefit, it is less profitable to work than to claim. For those on Family Income Supplement, if work is to be profitable, they must get a job earning £145 per week or more, which is often quite unrealistic. Claimants are therefore caught in the traps of poverty and unemployment.

In real life, the amounts paid out in benefits are inadequate to cover the basic necessities of life, and thus claimants often have no choice but to break the law, and to make some extra earnings 'on the side' in the black market. The annual turnover of the black economy in the UK has been estimated at some £36 billion. It is the fifth largest industry in the country, and all of its activities are of course untaxed. If even 1% of this activity could be coaxed back into the formal economy, GDP would increase by £360 000 000 and tax revenue by £72 000 000 (20% of £360 000 000). If amnesties were to be offered to those who are at present working in the black economy, at the same time as offering a way out of the poverty/unemployment traps, it is reasonable to expect that many would welcome the opportunity to step back into the legitimate world. The fear of being caught out is of itself a cause of stress and therefore illness. Some action must be taken: it cannot be in the best interests of the state to have up to 10% of its economically active citizens living outside of the law.

Unemployment and lawbreaking are therefore an inherent part of the present welfare state benefits system. This is an irrational and immoral state of affairs, especially when the financial, health and social costs of unemployment are counted. Citizen's Income, which simply removes the condition that to receive benefit a claimant must do no significant work, remedies this problem.

However, one of the stumbling blocks in the way of CI is that it appears to be both radical and expensive to conventional thinking. Computer models of the introduction of CI[13] show a high cost to the state because of the assumption that a large section of the workforce will choose not to work. Persuading public, press and politicians that this assumption is erroneous would cost time that we simply do not have: the crisis in social security is too urgent. For this reason, an alternative, gradual route to CI is presented here, introducing it as a form of wage subsidy that entirely sidesteps the above objection.

## Dead-end dole into wage subsidy

Ten per cent of the available workforce is suffering because they have no work to do. At the same time, there is a massive amount of necessary work waiting to be done in order to protect and improve our human and natural environment. Two problems, one solution: allow claimants to take their benefit to work with them when they find socially and environmentally beneficial work. In other words, the Treasury should stop applying 100% taxation to the benefit income of claimants when they begin work.

In fact, this is not a radical proposal. There are precedents in the current benefits system.

- Pensioners can earn on top of their pension.

- There is a measure in the Budget of April 1993 which allows those unemployed for more than two years to take employment and keep their benefit.
- There is also an 'earnings disregard' that allows a claimant to earn £2 per day or £12 per week over and above the benefit level of £44.65 (1993 levels).

These are all features akin to a CI, features that we can exploit to introduce new thinking in a manner that is painless to orthodox thinking.

Wage subsidy involves a small deletion of the available for work clause, but the implications for the economy are immense. Instead of being a dead dole, the benefit becomes a living and productive wage, an immense fillip to the real economy at no extra cost to the Treasury. True, the £25 billion annual cost of benefits remains, but it is turned into an investment in the creation of real wealth which will in due course repay the investment through increased tax take and many economic spin-offs.

Where new monies have to be found for capital expenditure associated with the new scheme, the government could exercise its power to create its own money to give out as low-interest loans (banks currently generate money out of nothing in the act of making loans). Whether by this means, or by more conventional borrowing, the fact remains that Keynesian investment in socially and ecologically beneficial work must be the way forward for the foundering economies of the UK and, indeed, the rest of the world.

## GREEN WORK

> Blessed is he who has found his work; let him ask no other blessedness.
>
> Thomas Carlyle

## Ecologically wised-up Keynesianism

Thomas Carlyle may have been going a bit over the top in this regard, but he does serve to remind us that there was a time when work was valued highly. Such statements are liable to be dismissed as the 'Protestant work ethic', but such derogatory labelling is no substitute for logical argument about the urgent need to reduce the entropy in the economic/ecological situation in which we find ourselves by carrying out a considerable amount of creative and constructive work.

The great British economist John Maynard Keynes argued that it was the duty of governments to lift the economy out of recession by providing money to invest in new work on the infrastructure of the country. Now that both communism and monetarism have demonstrably failed to meet the needs of people and environment, Keynesianism is coming back into its own; however, in the late twentieth century, Keynesian investment must be qualified and guided by ecological wisdom. Not all work creates real wealth. Arms production is an example of work that is highly profitable for the producer but which, overall, depletes the wealth of those who buy arms, and especially those who experience the end product in the flesh. The market economy needs to be guided into benign paths, both negatively, with taxes on products that are socially and environmentally harmful, and positively, by directing the wage subsidy to work that is beneficial to society and the environment.

Enterprises to benefit from wage subsidy labour should be:

- ecopositive (beneficial to the environment)
- socially positive (beneficial to the community)
- investment rather than simple expenditure
- labour intensive in preference to capital intensive.

Throughout this section, the word 'jobs' will be used as shorthand, while acknowledging that there is a large philosophical question over the value of paid employment as compared with non-alienated work.

## Introducing the wage subsidy

There is no suggestion of compulsion or 'workfare' in this proposal; people will take on work (or not, as the case may be) of their own free will, just as in the case of a citizen's income scheme, and no one who refuses work will be penalized in any way apart from the fact that they remain in status quo.

It has been objected that this scheme, since it is not a universal benefit, is not a bona fide citizen's income. This is true, but only in the sense that getting on a train is not the same thing as arriving at a destination. Transition is by definition a time of confusion, when two states overlap. The turnover in unemployment means that the number of jobs supported by wage subsidy will gradually increase. It has been found on the doorstep that the approach to a citizen's income, set out in this way, gains ready acceptance by the average citizen.

One of the most important advantages of this scheme is that it decreases labour costs, and it is precisely this factor that has resulted in the loss of industrial jobs to the tiger economies of the Pacific Rim: Japan, Korea, China and other countries with low wage bills. Wage subsidy means that British industry (and European, since it is likely that EU standardization rules mean the scheme will have to be implemented on a Europe-wide basis) will be able to compete on a more equal footing.

The increased economic activity generated by this scheme will pave the way in due course to implementation of full citizen's income. One pound in the pocket of the poor stimulates the economy seven times more than the same amount given to the rich, because the poor use the money in a way that feeds into the general economy faster, for instance in buying food or necessities. Money given to the rich tends to remain out of circulation as savings or to be exchanged for luxury items with other rich people.

In due course, as the stimulation of the economy works through to greater tax revenues, wage subsidy would be widened to include neutral service enterprises such as telephone cleaning; although arms manufacture, battery farming and road construction should never benefit from the scheme. As wage subsidy-generated wealth works through into the general economy, the scheme can be extended so that valuable enterprises needing extra support will receive subsidies for more of their workforce until all their employees are supported. Eventually the state will be able to make the final step (which at that stage would be quite small) into the unconditional universal benefit that is the citizen's income proper.

Constructive dialogue should be held with the unions to work out protocols and regulations to prevent newly subsidized labour from displacing those already in employment. This should not be difficult. Before wage subsidy labour joins the workforce, an employer will notify the existing number of employees to the Department of Employment, and will not be allowed to reduce that number while taking on new wage subsidy labour. This would need an inspectorate, but the work of the inspectors would be made easier by the fact that, in the event of displacement by wage subsidy labour, disgruntled displacees would be most likely to draw the inspectors' attention to their case, so that the system is self-regulating.

It should be pointed out to the unions that much of the proposed work is new, and will therefore pose no threat to existing jobs. Integration of the scheme with a minimum wage could be achieved with ease.

Activities in the Green sector often create redundancies in the non-Green sector – for instance, energy conservation will destroy work in nuclear energy production. Broadly speaking, however, Green work is more labour intensive than capital intensive, so that there will be a net gain.

## Stimulating the Green sector

The main areas to benefit will be the following:

- energy conservation
- renewable energy technologies
- energy-efficient goods manufacture
- pollution control technology
- waste minimization
- repair
- recycling
- water management
- sustainable agriculture
- forestry and timber use
- countryside management
- housing – new building and refurbishment
- the visual environment

- public transport
- education and training
- counselling, caring and healing
- community work
- leisure and tourism
- innovation, research and development
- any business that passes a certain threshold in its environmental audit.

In his paper *Growth, Employment and Environmental Policy*, Professor David Pearce[14] concluded that 'the evidence available does not support the received political wisdom that more environmental regulation will be harmful to economic growth'. He quotes Barker and Lewney,[15] who set the following scenario:

- carbon tax to attain 1990 levels of carbon dioxide output by 2005
- industrial pollution abatement spending quadrupled by 2000
- intensified water clean-up policy.

The Cambridge Multisectoral Dynamic model showed a fall in unemployment of 365 000 in 2005 compared with 1990 when this scenario was run.

Pearce also quotes an OECD study[16] which finds that 'employment is stimulated by the growth of the pollution abatement sector and a slight depressing effect on productivity'. These studies take a very narrow view of what is involved in 'greening' the economy. A more comprehensive view will turn up many more work opportunities. The next section investigates these opportunities sector by sector.

## Energy conservation

Our energy use has often been likened to a rich but stupid person trying to run a bath. Finding that it is filling slowly, he turns the tap on faster but fails to notice that the plug is not in the hole. Energy conservation is the equivalent of putting the plug in the hole. It is called demand-side management and, not unsurprisingly, has been found to be cheaper than supply-side management.[17] The Association for the Conservation of Energy[18] has calculated that a national programme of domestic energy conservation (loft and wall insulation, draughtproofing, heating controls and lighting efficiency) could create 500 000 job–years of work at a cost of £15.5 billion with a payback time of three to five years.

Out of this research came the Energy Conservation Bill, which was passed into law in early 1995 after humble beginnings as an early day motion by Plaid Cymru/Green MP Cynog Dafis, backed by a hard-fought campaign spearheaded by the Green Party but involving many environmental and social concern non-governmental organizations (NGOs) and gaining support from a majority of MPs of all parties. The campaign was won without any significant media coverage. The Energy Conservation Act requires local authorities to conduct an energy survey of all properties in their area and report on ways in which 'significant energy savings' can be achieved, with the financial costs and the resultant reduction in carbon dioxide output documented. There will be a statement of the council's policy for taking into account the 'personal circumstances' (e.g. poverty, age, disability) of households surveyed. The Secretary of State for the Environment must set times for reports and reviews to come back, and has indicated that they will seek a 30% reduction initially. They must assist councils with resourcing the Act, and must report back to parliament on progress.

The Energy Conservation Act offsets the increased cost to the low paid that resulted from the introduction of VAT on fuel by reducing the amount of fuel that is used. The cost-effectiveness of the measure is increased by reducing housing maintenance costs by approximately £100–£500 per annum per dwelling as a result of the reduction in dampness in houses.

All new jobs have a 'multiplier effect' as the new wages are spent on goods and services. Jobs created in energy efficiency have an additional 'respender' effect, as money saved on energy is respent on goods and services. The costs per job per year have been variously estimated at between £9000 and £23 000. At the lower end of the range, the job comes free of cost to the state if the worker is taken from the dole. As with all Green energy measures, jobs created in the Green sector will displace jobs in finite fuel industries. Tables in *Working Future?*[6] show that, for every job lost, three are gained.

For the estimate here, we will take as a minimum the lower figure from *Working Future?*[6] of 36 000 and as a maximum the ACE report figure of 500 000 job–years, which, if spread over ten years, give 50 000 jobs per year.

## Renewable energy technologies

The manufacture, installation and maintenance of renewable energy technology – wind turbines, wave energy devices, biomass systems, solar heat systems, fuel cells, photovoltaic systems, auxiliary sails for commercial ships and others – will clearly become a major industry in the future, and in order to secure the UK a niche in the future market it is vital to make a start now, reversing the government inaction and hostility that have lost us the initiative in the development of wave and wind power.

The European Wind Energy Association has published a report, *Wind Energy in Europe – A Plan of Action.*[19] The report stated that large employment gains were not expected from any programme of renewable energy, no matter how ambitious, because for each job created in renewables a job will be lost from the fossil energy sector. The point was also made that lead times for wind energy installations are considerably less than those for fossil and nuclear stations. In addition, wind turbine systems, once in place, need remarkably little maintenance. Labour needs are limited to an attendant to keep a general eye on the site.

However, the FoE report[6] gives a different picture, with wind power of 30 TWh/year creating 6900–13 800 jobs or 3420–10 320 when displacement of coal work is accounted for. A maximum effort to harness all available onshore wind could create up to 55 000 jobs.

Germany is commencing an ambitious solar energy scheme using roof tiles with built-in photovoltaic cells which generate electricity for storage. This scheme could be developed here: no estimate has been made for the work created.

It is estimated that a combined heat and power scheme, where waste heat is piped around housing estates, would provide 140 000 job–years for only five cities, or 7000–12 000 jobs over 15 years, taking into account job displacement.

## Energy-efficient goods manufacture

This is certainly a Green enterprise, but cannot be counted on as a means of job creation since it will simply displace jobs in inefficient manufacture. However, it merits inclusion, since if the UK persists in opting out of incoming EU energy standards (as occurred in the matter of energy-efficient domestic gas boiler manufacture) we will lose both export and domestic markets to superior EU goods. The use of energy-efficient goods benefits the economy as it reduces fuel poverty as well as global warming.

# Pollution control technologies

Pollution control constitutes the most common Green technology proposal in academic assessments that have been carried out. A Labour Party study[20] showed 628 000 jobs would be created by increasing environmental standards. Cambridge Econometrics[21] calculated that 200 000 jobs would be created by a faithful application of the polluter pays principle, and 696 000 from a major investment in improving water quality.

Technologies for the recapture and re-use of solid, liquid and gaseous 'waste' materials exist in many forms, but in order to reach the market place they need environmental legislation that is strictly enforced. Despite the lack of such a legislative ethos in the UK, there is a healthy export market for British-produced water pollution control equipment.

# Waste minimization

Project Catalyst was an initiative in the Wirral that aimed to reduce waste in industry. The project covered 14 companies, at a cost of £1 million, and came up with savings worth £2 million a year that would continue to accrue while the processes ran. Simply ordering their suppliers to cut a rubber door seal to the right size saved one firm £20 000 per year and many skiploads of six-inch rubber offcuts. This project is a classic case to justify government investment in industrial and environmental efficiency. It will not necessarily create jobs, but by increasing the prosperity of firms could make existing jobs more secure.

In a review of the initiative[22] by the Department of Trade and Industry the numbers of employees in the firm and the annual financial value of the saving is given in 12 cases. From these figures an index of money saved per annum per employee (PAPE) can be derived. It varied from £46 to £6842, with an arithmetical average of £1568. Extrapolation of this figure to the numbers employed in all industry in September 1993 (5 359 000) gives a crude estimate of annual savings of £8 402 912 000 (£8.4 billion) per year to be obtained from waste minimization, which is, as the Prime Minister would say, a not inconsiderable sum.

# Repair

If resource taxes are brought in, together with other disincentives designed to discourage the 'disposable' mentality, repair of defective goods will once again become an important activity. Although this will mean some job losses in manufacturing industries, there should be a net gain since repair is more labour intensive than assembly line manufacture because of the extra time spent dismantling the article – it has been estimated that 56% more labour is needed to recondition a motor car than to build it from scratch.[23]

In order to give this factor some quantitative representation, an increase in manufacturing jobs will be assumed. Taking 1–5% of the number of manufacturing jobs in 1993 of 4 million as a base gives 40 000 to 200 000.

# Recycling

Recycling is commonly seen as an activity of marginal economic significance. This is erroneous. In 1983 imports of paper to the UK were worth more than the UK's entire motor car export market. Recycling of paper to an extent that would reduce these imports to zero should therefore be seen as equally important as the objective of doubling our exports of cars.

Kerbside collections and manual sorting (as opposed to mechanical sorting systems) are highly labour-intensive operations. Cardiff, Milton Keynes, Leeds, Bath and Bristol all have a variety of systems of kerbside collection for waste.

In Bath there is a weekly pick-up of recyclable goods. Workers segregate the waste on the pick-up vehicle. Eight people are directly employed in collecting and sorting, and they cover 14 000 households (ratio of workers to households = 1:1750). Cardiff, with a similar scheme, has 30 people serving 128 000 households (ratio = 1:4264).

Although these schemes operate in cities, there is no reason why they should not also operate successfully in the countryside. Recycling, segregating pick-ups can also be integrated into the routine waste collection.

Scaling these ratios up to cover the whole of the UK would create between 5624 and 13 000 jobs in collection alone. Since this is hard physical work, with an element of danger attached to it, it would be better to choose the more labour-intensive option of 13 000 jobs.

More work is needed at the depots in processing the recycled waste. Assuming one reprocessing job to ten collecting jobs, this gives another 1300 places.

More work will be created at the plant where the recycled materials are reintroduced into the manufacturing stream, but since these will displace jobs in manufacturing from virgin resources their input will be assumed to be zero.

This crude estimate of between 6924 and 14 300 jobs in recycling compares reasonably well with the estimates quoted in *Working Future?*[6] of 7200 and 8500 jobs in recycling paper and returnable drinks containers.

## Water management

The quality of drinking water supply needs improving in many ways. The first priority must be to replace domestic lead piping, especially in soft-water areas, since long-term ingestion of low levels of lead is known to cause lowering of intelligence in children. Seventy per cent of the piping that needs replacement lies in the curtilage of the dwelling, so that grants for replacement must be made available for families on low income. Wage subsidy support will reduce labour costs substantially for this work on higher incomes, but further direct subsidies should support the work in order to reduce the financial disincentive for this preventive health measure.

The quantity of drinking water supplies is restricted in droughts, which will become more frequent as global warming progresses. About 30% of the UK water supply is lost through leaking mains. Leaks also present the threat of contamination of the supply if mains pressure falls below the pressure of water in the surrounding soil, which may in turn be contaminated with leakage from adjoining sewers. There is therefore a case for major investment in mains renewals. Unfortunately in the privatized water industry more investment means less dividend for shareholders and less rakeoff for the chairmen. It has not been possible to get an estimate for the numbers of jobs which would be created in this programme.

Sewerage refurbishment is already in hand, forced by the advanced state of decay of Victorian sewers. The costs of the work will be repaid by avoiding the inconvenience of the sudden appearance of large holes in the street. Sewer collapses are commonly measured in units called DDBs, one DDB being a hole large enough to swallow a double decker bus. A further health and aesthetic benefit comes from a reduction in the rate of increase of the rat population. Rats use sewers as routes of expansionary migration, escaping upwards to new territories through cracks and gaps in the old brickwork.

New sewerage networks are required for industrial waste water management in order to end the practice of mixing industrial wastes and domestic sewage. Without this, treated sludges cannot safely and sustainably be recycled to land because of the build-up of industry-derived heavy metals and other toxins in the soil. This might create an estimated 5000 jobs per year for ten years.

Biodigestion is the process by which organic wastes such as sewage and vegetation are broken down by bacteria, into simpler, homogenized and non-toxic end products that can then be re-used. Various forms exist from the common or garden compost heap through anaerobic digestion to a new process where by a micro-organism derived from horse dung effectively causes the slow oxidation of the waste, producing heat and carbon dioxide gas.

Biodigestion is the jewel in the crown of Green technologies. It can turn sewage, a foul and hazardous waste product that emits methane and ammonia (both greenhouse gases) into energy-producing gas (or low-grade heat) and an enhanced organic fertilizer that meshes with the needs of the organic farmer. Farm Gas plc claims that the energy value alone can pay back the cost of installation in two years. Unfortunately, however, owing to the lack of encouragement from either subsidies or regulation, the commercial exploitation of biodigestion is languishing in the UK, in contrast to Denmark, where the proportion of sewage treated in this way is approaching 100%.

Employment opportunities in biodigestion would arise in the manufacture of digesters and also in maintenance. There is also the matter of the export market, and this is a technology *par excellence* that could be transferred to developing countries under the Rio proposals for transfer of benign technologies. It is a pity that most of the export credit guarantees that support British exports are applied to armaments rather than benign technologies such as biodigestion.

Water management includes:

- improvement of habitat of wildlife around waterways
- rehabilitation, commercial and leisure use of canals
- sea defences.

Coastal erosion is a serious problem in many sites around the UK. The emerging thinking on the subject is that things should be allowed to slide (literally), and this may be wise in many sites, given the conspicuous failure of King Canute. In some sites, however, the use of wave power barrages may be a useful and cost-effective solution to beach erosion. The Ministry for Agriculture, Fisheries and Food (MAFF) has been urged to consider that in some sites wave energy barrages might be used to defend the coast and to build up the beaches. The Lanchester barrage is known to be able to do this. The counter-argument has been that erosion damage occurs during storms, and storm waves would simply sweep over wave devices. This is true, but if the beach were built up by the presence of the barrage the storm energy would expend itself on the beach, as it has always done, and as it does on beaches everywhere, rather on farm land, as occurs when the beach has been eroded. The idea of using wave power in this way has not been ruled out by MAFF and it has been agreed that more research is needed. For the scheme to be developed would need more coordination between government departments than is the case at present, and also a less hostile attitude towards wave power than has been shown hitherto by government.

For a crude estimate of the increase in numbers available under the wage subsidy scheme, let us assume that the National Rivers Authority, which presently has 7500 employees increases its staff five to ten per cent, i.e. 375–750.

Flood control is necessary to prevent intermittent flooding of certain vulnerable valleys. Flooding certainly causes much financial and emotional hardship to those who are flooded, and a case might be made for investing in flood prevention. However, the environmental impact of flood prevention work needs very careful and critical assessment. Left to themselves, rivers naturally flood from time to time. Confining a river between narrow banks may in some circumstances simply displace the flood further downriver, and may also alter the natural ecosystem.

Building river levees was one of the key works in the New Deal in the USA, and many of the results were not good for the environment. Nevertheless, there may be a case for identifying sites where flood prevention works might be ecologically acceptable.

The job count for water pollution control has been mentioned earlier (p. 47) at 696 000.

## Sustainable agriculture

Employment in rural areas has been falling inexorably as a result of the mechanization of agriculture. Small farmers are depressed both economically and emotionally. According to Richard Young, an organic farmer, demand for labour is slightly higher in organic farming than conventional farming in the areas of animal husbandry (reflecting better care) and weeding organic fields, but this is offset by labour savings in spraying. He estimates the labour requirements of wheat growing per acre to be equal for organic and chemical farmers. However, he goes on to state, 'It would not be that difficult to build a case showing that organic farmers use substantially more labour per unit of food'. Here is the case:

- set-aside removes 15% of land from production
- this will cause the collapse of smaller farmers and 'will concentrate power in the larger farms and lead to another cranking up of the intensification spiral ... more tractors mean less [people]'
- fifteen per cent less land in production will therefore lead to more than 15% fewer employees
- organic yields are on average 26% lower than intensive yields
- the objective of set-aside (reduced production in the EU to reduce the food mountains) could therefore be achieved by an increase in organic production without the loss of 15% of the workforce.

Nick Lampkin's book *Organic Farming in Practice*[24] reproduces a table in which the labour requirement of organic farms and conventional farms is compared and is found (coincidentally) to be 15% higher for organic farms. However, Lampkin gives a number of reasons that these estimates cannot be transferred directly to the

British farming scene. He concludes, 'Organic farming is often associated with increased labour use.'

According to *Working Future?*[6] 30 000–40 000 extra jobs would be created as a result of a 25% conversion to organic or sustainable agriculture.

## Gardening and allotment cultivation

Gardening and allotment cultivation are an important part of sustainable agriculture. Gardening is one of the most efficient ways of producing food. Wage subsidy could increase the availability of workers willing to cultivate the gardens of elderly people on a share-cropping basis. This could improve the diet of people in deprived areas.

Let us assume that 0.1% of 4 million unemployed, i.e. 4000, become active full time in this form of cultivation.

## Ecologically sound forestry and timber use

The *Forestry Industry Yearbook 1992–93*[25] gives the number of people directly employed in forestry as 41 050, with approximately 540 000 employed in industries that use timber – pulp and paper manufacture and furniture manufacture and distribution. The activity that contributes the largest amount to the employment total is harvesting. Forestry employment is predicted to rise from 41 050 to 60 000 by the year 2001 as the trees planted in the 1940s are harvested, and towards 66 000 in 2006, although higher productivity through mechanization might reduce this figure to 48 000. Let us assume that wage subsidy gives a 5–10% boost to this figure, i.e. creates 2400–4800 extra jobs.

In fact this estimate could be extremely conservative. Irvine[26] advocates the 'forest farm' concept of ecologically sound forestry. This involves a move away from mechanization and chemical forestry management and therefore away from high productivity assumptions, towards high labour input.[27,28]

An interesting and pleasing link exists between the solution to global warming and the demand for fine craftsmanship. As the perception that wood has a special value as a solidified form of carbon dioxide percolates into the public consciousness, wood will be increasingly valued as a structural material. The longer a wooden object is kept, the longer that carbon dioxide will remain locked up. One way of ensuring that an object is kept is to subject it to fine craftsmanship. Therefore, woodworkers of all kinds should be favoured by the programme, with bonuses apportioned according to aesthetic quality. Let us assume that 500–1000 new workers in this field result from wage subsidy encouragement.

## Countryside management programmes

The Department of the Environment (DoE) has published a brochure, *Action for the Countryside*,[29] which provides a useful overview of the problems and policies. It also points to the Countryside Employment Programme, which comprises three pilot projects – primarily training, reskilling, and business advice and support.

At present, English Nature employs 846 people in an advisory capacity, the Countryside Council in Wales employs 320, the Countryside Commission 150 and the British Trust Conservation Volunteers (BTCV) 300 – 1616 in all. The BTCV uses in excess of 84 000 volunteers on a part-time basis.

Even the most casual walker can see to what extent the land created work in the past, when dry stone walls stretch for miles out into what is now 'empty' hill-side. The scope for work in clearing rubbish, laying hedges, upgrading footpaths, improving amenity and habitats is vast. People's enjoyment of the countryside, and therefore the national 'feelgood factor', would be enhanced as a result of these works.

In addition, Community Service labour could be used to carry out heavy and arduous work that might otherwise be of marginal economic value, such as col-lecting a proportion (some must be left to stimulate fungal growth) of fallen trees for sale as firewood. Community Service is in any case many times more cost-effective as a way of repaying convicts' debt to society than imprisonment.

Let us assume that the extra numbers of wage subsidy workers on the land would be between 1600 (equal to the numbers in the quangos above) and 8400 (10% of the volunteers used).

## Housing

Shelter has published a paper, *Homes cost less than Homelessness*,[30] which argues that the country could save £174 million per annum by building enough houses for the homeless instead of paying for them to live in bed and breakfast, hotels and leased property. These options cost £11 000–£13 000 per annum per family, whereas the cost of borrowing to build a council house is £7000 per annum according to Shelter's accounting convention, which takes into account the annual cost of repaying the home loan. However, the government insists that the full cost of paying for the home should be met in the year in which the home is built, which makes the cost of building appear prohibitively expensive. The government also ignores the fact that a home can produce an income (rent).

As well as building new houses to meet housing needs, especially in the social housing sector, there is a great deal of potential work available in the refurbish-ment of existing housing stock.

Since 1989, over 500 000 construction workers have lost their jobs.[31] Shelter's proposals for boosting the stock by 100 000 units of social housing would generate employment for 120 000 people.[32] It calls for £1.3 billion per year for five years (£6.5 billion) to be spent in refurbishment and new building. Already £5.5 billion is held in local authority funds from the sale of council houses, so only another £1 billion will have to be found, which would be repaid in 5.7 years from the savings in temporary accommodation of £174 million per year mentioned above. Every £1 billion invested in new housing creates 50 000 jobs, so that at least 250 000 job–years will be created. This will be counted as 50 000 per year from 1997 to 2002.

## Improvements to the visual environment

Depressed people see the world as lifeless, grey and ugly. Conversely, a lifeless, grey and ugly environment can only be expected to make people depressed and alienated. Both social and economic paybacks are therefore to be expected from a programme of tidying, cleaning, painting and planting in public spaces. This is already happening to a certain extent (for instance with the Thames bridges in London), but we should be seeking to bring the amenity usually reserved for areas of tourist attraction into the environment of the average citizen.

As well as a general increase in happiness and productivity, there are material gains to be had from a painting programme: wood and iron structures will benefit from a prolongation of their useful lives because of the protective effects of paint.

Oscar Wilde was quite wrong when he said that all art is quite useless. At a rough estimate, assuming that each of 500 district councils employed about 50 people in this scheme, the net gain would be about 25 000 permanent jobs.

## Expansion of public transport services

Public transport work will comfortably offset the lay-offs that Green policies will cause in the motor car and road construction industry. The cheaper labour brought about by wage subsidy will enable conductors and porters to return, making public transport user-friendlier and safer, since the reintroduction of conductors will reduce the fear of violence from other passengers. Pollution and journey times will also be reduced as the bus will not stand for so long while the driver collects the fares.

Friends of the Earth, working from statistics in a Worldwatch report,[33] estimated the effects of transferring from road construction work to work in rail, rail freight and light railways (Table 3.2).

Transferral labour is needed to move freight from lorries to rail. At the moment, it is the high cost of this labour that is responsible for putting so much freight on the roads. Wage subsidy labour could reduce these costs, pending a longer term solution involving raising the height of train tunnel roofs in order to allow the trailer part of articulated lorries to be loaded directly on to rail trucks for long journeys. The Channel Tunnel has made the use of rail for international freight journeys potentially far more economical, since it avoids the need for freight to be transferred from rail to ferry and back again.

**Table 3.2** Number of jobs created by transferring labour from road construction

|  | Jobs estimate | |
| --- | --- | --- |
|  | Low | High |
| £500 million transferred to rail and rail freight | 3 000 | 8 150 |
| £400 million transferred to light rail | 3 475 | 7 590 |
| Total | 6 475 | 15 740 |

**Table 3.3**  Cost of creating cycleways

| Cost per kilometre of cycleway | £000s |
|---|---|
| Painted lines on quiet backstreet | 1 |
| Pavement conversion for shared use | 5–15 |
| Virgin cycleway | 25–40 |

Cycleways, together with traffic restraint and integrated transport policies, are a necessary part of breaking the motor car habit. The cost of creating cycleways varies with the topography of the area and to what extent the cycleway stands alone or is part of another scheme (Table 3.3).

Cycleways are built to a high specification in order to last, usually by contractors who make roads. Cycleways could therefore compensate for lost opportunities in road construction, but whereas a job in roadbuilding costs about £70 000, it is estimated that two jobs building cycleways could be created for that sum.

Sustrans, which campaigns for and builds cycleways, has a plan to build an 8000-km cycleway in the UK over ten years. Taking a mean figure of £30 000 per kilometre to allow for the fact that some of the work is in cities and therefore cheaper, this gives an overall cost of £240 million, and if each £35 000 creates one job the total job count is 6857 over the ten years, or 690 per year.

## Education and training programmes

Money put into education is an investment in the future of the nation, and this alone is enough to justify an increase in the numbers employed in education. There are 392 900 teachers in nursery, primary and secondary education in the UK. They teach in classes with pupil–teacher ratios of up to and over 30:1, and the available evidence shows that the quality of education improves with smaller class sizes.

For instance, research in Tennessee reported in June 1995 that children in classes of under 15 fared better at reading and writing than those in classes of 25. Half of the extra cost was recouped from savings in remedial teaching, and the other half is expected to be recouped in increased taxes from the better educated children when they enter work.

There are 53 256 teachers in local education authority further education colleges, excluding those controlled by polytechnics and colleges of further education. If a programme of retraining led to a 5–10% increase in these positions, an additional 2663–5326 jobs in training would be created.

To reduce from class sizes of 30:1 to 20:1 would call for a 50% increase in the establishment of education nationally or, say, an extra 150 000 permanent jobs.

## Counselling, caring and health work

There is evidence that these activities represent excellent investment from both a humanitarian and financial standpoint.

A report commissioned by Relate[34] concluded that the service it provides saves the state more than £42.8 million per annum through savings in Legal Aid, Family Support and other indirect costs of divorce. The cost to the state of funding Relate's services is £2.2 million, mostly paid by local authorities. Relate considers that its work in the UK could be expanded by a factor of ten. This is clearly a very efficient use of public money.

Active working counsellors at Relate at present number 2669; so 28 000 extra jobs could be added through a tenfold expansion of its services.

Parenthood counselling is likewise an excellent investment in the future. Assuming that each counsellor can sustain a caseload of 50 and that 1% of Britain's households with children need counselling leads to the following figures.

| | |
|---|---|
| UK population | 57 million |
| UK households @ 2.4 each | 23.75 million |
| 48% of households have children | 11.4 million |
| 1% need counselling | 114 000 |
| 50 per counsellor | 2280 counsellors |

Similar numbers might be required for other special groups: for adolescents, drug and alcohol abusers and so on. The demand for counsellors is likely to be limited only by the ability of existing counsellors to train new workers.

Carers for sick family or neighbours must undergo a stringent bureaucratic procedure to qualify for financial aid. Wage subsidy would make this procedure much easier.

Formal caring, for instance community care of people with learning difficulties or mental illness or children in care, is labour-intensive work. Social service group workers should have a staffing ratio of at least one worker to five service users; however, increased ratios would lead to higher quality work, and in children's homes the ratio should be 1:1. The inspectorate for nursing homes and residential homes of all kinds should also be increased, with irregular unscheduled visits to ensure that standards are maintained and that no abuses occur.

The NHS is the biggest single employer in the UK, with a workforce standing at 211 000 in 1991. This is down from 214 000 in 1988, but roughly equivalent to the staffing levels in 1981. Overwork and personnel shortages are constant complaints from health workers in every sector. A 1% increase in care workers as a result of wage subsidy would yield 21 400 new jobs, and a 0.1% increase would yield 2140 jobs.

## Community work

Community workers whose aim is to catalyse the coming together of people to discover the strength that exists in working together are known to be able to benefit society. If it is assumed that 10% of households (2.375 million) could benefit from this kind of input, and that each worker could serve 100 households, we have a need for 23 750 community workers.

## Leisure and tourism

New patterns of work and the ability of machines to take over much repetitive work means that we will all have more leisure time. Already there is growth in quantity and quality of the leisure industry. Any constructive and healthy use of leisure time should be encouraged with wage subsidy.

## Innovation, research and development

Although not directly a source of mass employment, indirectly a successful pro- gramme of innovation, research and development will benefit the economy. Any shift of the economy towards truly sustainable development predicates innovation. Before 1994, the Department of Trade and Industry's Design Council ran a Noticeboard Project that assessed innovations, advised innovators on the presenta- tion of their projects and put details of successful ideas before the related sections of industry. This should be reinstated, and consideration should be given to the question of making loans to facilitate the early stages of innovation. Many innova- tions are lost through the lack of money (beginning at £1000–£2000) required during the difficult inception period.

## Environmentally and socially friendly businesses

Any company or business that passes an environmental audit to a certain standard should be able to qualify for wage subsidy support. Environmental audit should involve a survey of the business consumption of resources, its output product, its wastes and their effect and working conditions within the business. The prospect of being able to benefit from wage subsidy would stimulate interest in minimizing waste, producing useful and durable products and optimizing working conditions.

The total employment creation opportunity through carrying out necessary work is summarized in Table 3.4.

# How is it all to be paid for?

## There is no alternative

It is beyond the scope of this book to carry out the detailed quantitative projec- tions for the wage subsidy scheme. Between 1.3 and 2 million full-time jobs have been identified by the method outlined above. The work is not work for its own sake, but serious and vitally necessary from the point of view of sustainable devel- opment. In many cases, for example in housebuilding, energy conservation and marriage guidance counselling, there is a clearly identifiable financial payback. In other cases, for instance sustainable agriculture, improvements to the visual envi- ronment and in forestry, there is an ecological payback but the financial paybacks will not be clear until an index of sustainable economic welfare supplants the old, crude measure of GNP.

**Table 3.4** Jobs gained through 'greening' the economy (estimate)

| Estimate | 000s | |
|---|---|---|
| | High | Low |
| Taxing resources, not jobs | 150 | 278 |
| Cambridge Multisectoral Dynamic model | 365 | 365 |
| Energy efficiency[a] | 50 | 36 |
| Wind onshore | 50 | 18 |
| Active solar[b] | 1 | 1 |
| Combined heat and power (CHP) | 12.5 | 7.9 |
| Pollution control | 696 | 200 |
| Repair | 200 | 40 |
| Recycling | 14.3 | 6.9 |
| Sewerage | 5 | 5 |
| Waterways | 0.75 | 0.375 |
| Sustainable agriculture | 40 | 30 |
| Gardening/allotments | 4 | 4 |
| Forestry, expected | 48 | 48 |
| Forestry, wage subsidy added | 4.8 | 2.4 |
| Fine wood craftsmanship | 1 | 0.1 |
| Countryside management | 8.4 | 1.6 |
| Housebuilding for five years | 50 | 50 |
| Painting and decorating | 25 | 25 |
| Transfer from road to rail | 15.74 | 6.48 |
| Cycleways | 0.69 | 0.69 |
| Teachers | 150 | 150 |
| Trainers | 5.33 | 2.66 |
| Relate counsellors | 28 | 28 |
| Parental counsellors | 2 | 2 |
| Community workers | 23.8 | 23.8 |
| NHS | 21.4 | 2.14 |
| Ban on tobacco advertising (see page 167) | 1.87 | 1.87 |
| Total | 1 974.580 | 1 336.915 |

[a] displacement corrected
[b] displacement corrected

The effect of wage subsidy is that Social Security Benefit expenditure, instead of being money thrown away on a process that condemns people to exist in a state of surly and impecunious idleness, is converted into a surge of financial and human energy into the economy which, if wisely directed towards improving the ecological infrastructure of the economy, can resolve two of the major challenges of our time: the pain of unemployment and poverty and the threat of ecological collapse.

A simple example of what is needed exists in Beira, Mozambique. There the water table is high, so that puddles form easily. Mosquitoes breed in the water and cause malaria, which imposes a huge strain on the health services. Standing by the puddles are crowds of unemployed people, and behind them is sand. What is required is to use the unemployed to fill the puddles with sand. The authorities know this, but because their country has been bled dry by 20 years of war, they have no money to pay for the work to be done. Monetarists would say that this is as it should be: they must wait for the money to come along. Keynesians would say that the government should borrow money to carry out the necessary work, and pay it back when times are less hard.

Some economists go further than Keynes: they point out that the money is borrowed from banks, and that the banks neither borrow to fund the loan nor draw on their reserves: they lend virtual money, created from nothing.

If a person requests a loan from a bank, the bank manager assesses the financial credibility of the person. If the person is of good standing, and the purpose of the loan is reasonable, the manager grants it. The only limit on the bank's ability to lend is the surety provided by the capital sums in the bank's vaults: total loans must not exceed a certain multiple of what the bank holds. When a loan has been made, it is repaid many times over by the borrower earning the money in the real world by making real (or perhaps relatively real) objects. By drawing in these real earnings, the bank's assets are increased, so that even more virtual money can be lent in years to come.

Some economists question why this alchemical power should be delegated solely to the banks, and why it should not be exercised, with due caution and safeguards, by governments and even communities. Chief among the safeguards is that there should be a reasonable expectation of a payback, which is the case in the areas outlined above.

In short, lack of money should not stop the Beirans from filling their puddles, nor should it stop us from filling our own social and environmental puddles. Money exists to serve the real economy; the economy does not exist to serve money. If real ecopositive work needs to be done, money should be created against the surety of the physical and human resources available, and against the soundness of the plan. This money creation is not inflationary since the end result is an increase in the total value within the system. At the end of the day, it must be better to get the unemployed working on good constructive projects than paying them a semi-adequate subsistence pittance on condition that they do no work.

## A balance sheet

The only accurate way to show that the wage subsidy will work is by running it on a computer model of the economy that can account for the dynamic effect of the influx of work into the economy, as well as the effects of improved general morale. In the absence of the use of such a program, the alternative is to present a simple arithmetical calculation to show that it is possible to balance the books.

The balance sheet: gross cost of creating 2 million jobs by wage subsidy:

|  | £ billion |
|---|---|
| 1.0 million will be @ £8000 per year | 8 |
| 0.5 million will be @ £12 000 per year | 6 |
| 0.5 million will be @ £16 000 per year | 8 |
| Total | £22 billion |

From this figure, subtract the cost of removing 2 million from the dole at £9000 each (£18 billion). This leaves an extra £4 billion to be found. While it is true that a substantial part of the £18 billion will yet have to be paid (some administrative savings may be available), this money would have been paid out anyway, in dead-end dole money, and so can be discounted in this exercise which is to meet the extra costs.

| State savings per year | £ million |
|---|---|
| Wages bill for 2 million new jobs | (2000) |
| GNP increases by 2% | 12 000 |
| Building houses | 174 |
| Counselling | 360 |
| Waste minimization | 8403 |
| Axe allowance on company cars | 2000 |
| Collect unclaimed tax | 5000 |
| Axe Trident | 2000 |
| Total | 27 937 |

Even if the £18 billion wage subsidy is included in this equation, the country is still £9 937 000 000 (nearly 10 billion pounds) per year better off.

To this calculation can be added the fact that there is plenty of scope for increased borrowing in the UK. To restore the general level of investment in the UK to 1979 levels would require an annual increase of £22.5 billion.[10] Furthermore, if it is argued that, in spite of the savings outlined above, an increase in borrowing or taxation is needed, the predictable shock-horror reaction would not be supported by international comparisons. Projections by the OECD for 1996 indicate that Britain's annual government takings will amount to 37.9% of GDP, as opposed to the European average of 45.2%. Of EU countries, only Greece has a lower tax requirement than Britain. Similarly, Britain's borrowing projections for the year 2000 are only 47.4% of GDP, compared with an European average of 70%.

The conclusion is that, with a few minor adjustments to the spending programme, the country could comfortably afford to get back to work. If, in spite of all, the wage subsidy (or outright citizen's income) scheme is dismissed as too much out of line with accepted thinking, then society still has a decision. The poor, as Jesus said, are always with us. In addition, the unemployed are also with us. Full employment in its classic sense is a thing of the past. It is not sustainable to carry on as we are, grudgingly carrying those for whom we have no economic role in the present system, giving them a pittance to keep them from starving on condition that they do no work, and snatching it back if they do find work. Either government creates a rational welfare system that works along the lines outlined above or it creates workfare, work camps and finally extermination camps for those who are superfluous to current economic requirements, in the manner pioneered by Hitler. And in case any right-wing reader thinks that this is a serious proposition, let it be said now that such a solution would lead to exactly the same mayhem and destruction that Hitler caused. We cannot go down that path; we cannot remain where we are: therefore we have no option but to go for citizen's income by way of wage subsidy.

# REFERENCES

1    Turnbull C (1963) *The Forest People.* The Reprint Society with Chatto and Windus, London.

2    Lawson R (1991) *Green Policies in a Nutshell.* Woodspring Green Party.

3    New Economics Foundation: (e-mail: neweconomics@gn.apc.org), 1st floor, Vine Court, 112–116 Whitechapel Road, London.

4    Brundtland Report (1987) *Our Common Future. Brundtland Commission.* Oxford University Press, Oxford.

5    Pearce D (1993) *Blueprint 3: Measuring Sustainable Development.* Earthscan, London.

6    Friends of the Earth (1994) *Working Future? Jobs and the Environment.* FoE, London.

7    Piachaud D (1994) A Price Worth Paying? The cost of mass unemployment. *Economic Report Vol. 8, No. 6.* Employment Policy Institute, London.

8    Ecology Party (1982) *Working for a Future: An Ecological Approach to Employment.* Ecology Party, London.

9    Friends of the Earth (1994) *Working Future. Jobs and the Environment.* Friends of the Earth discussion paper. Friends of the Earth, London.

10   Fryer D and Payne R (1984) Proactive behaviour in unemployment: findings and implications. *Leisure Stud.* **3**; 273–95.

11   Robertson J (1994) *Benefits and Taxes: A Radical Strategy.* New Economics Foundation, London.

12   Bureau de Plan – Erasme (1993) In: A Majocchi (ed.) *The Employment effects of Eco-taxes: a review of empirical models and results.* Paper presented at the OECD Workshow on Implementation of Environmental Taxes, Paris, February 1994.

13   The Netherlands Central Planning Bureau (1994) Paper presented to the Fifth Biennial Congress of the Basic Income European Network. London, September.

**14**   Pearce D (1991) Growth, Employment and Environmental Policy. *Economic Report: 6(1)*. Employment Institute, London.

**15**   Barker T and Lewney R (1991) A Green scenario for the UK economy. In: T Barker (ed.) *Green Futures for Economic Growth: Britain in 2010*. Cambridge Econometrics, Cambridge.

**16**   OECD (1985) *The Macroeconomic Impact of Environmental Expenditure*. OECD, Paris.

**17**   Krier B and Goodman I (1993) *Energy Efficiency: Opportunities for Employment*. Greenpeace UK, London.

**18**   Taylor L (1993) *Enquiry into the Employment Impact of Investment in Energy Conservation*. For House of Commons Employment Select Committee, London.

**19**   European Wind Energy Association (1991) *Wind Energy in Europe – A Plan of Action*. Rome.

**20**   Labour Party (1994) Labour Party Commission on the Environment. In: *Trust for Tomorrow*. Labour Party, London.

**21**   Barker T and Lewney R (1990) Macroeconomic Modelling of Environmental Policies: The Carbon Tax, the Polluter Pays Principle and Regulation of Water Quality. In: T Barker (ed.) *A Green Scenario for the UK Economy*. Cambridge Econometrics, Cambridge.

**22**   Department of Trade and Industry (1992) *Cutting your Losses. A Further Guide to Waste Minimization for Business*. Department of Trade and Industry, London.

**23**   Stahel W R and Jackson T (1993) Optimal Utilisation and Durability. In: *Clean Production Strategies*. Lewis Publishers, London. pp. 261–94.

**24**   Lampkin N (1990) *Organic Farming*. Farming Press Books, Ipswich.

**25**   The Forestry Industry Council of Great Britain (1994) *The Forestry Industry Yearbook 1992–1993*. FICGB, London.

**26**   Irvine S and Ponton A (1993) *Woodman Spare that Tree!* Real World Publishing, Newcastle.

**27**   Land Use Working Group (1989) *A Rural Manifesto for the Highlands. Creating the Second Great Wood of Caledon*. Green Party, Highland, Inverness.

**28**   Reforest the Earth Campaign (1992) *UK Forest Charter and Demands*. Manifesto, Norwich.

**29**   Department of the Environment (1992) *Action for the Countryside*. Department of the Environment, London.

**30**   Walentowicz P (1992) *Homes cost less than Homelessness*. Shelter, London.

**31**   Building Employer's Confederation. Personal communication.

**32**   Shelter (1993) *Supply 100 000 homes, create jobs*. Shelter, London.

**33**   Renner M (1992) Creating Sustainable jobs in Industrial Countries. In: *State of the World*. Worldwatch Institute, Earthscan, London. pp. 138–54.

**34**  Compass Partnership (1990) *The Public Cost of Separation and Divorce and the Cost–Benefit of Relate's Work.* 10 Barley Mow Passage, London.

# 4

# The impact of poor housing on health[b]

*Interviewer: Mr Gandhi, what do you think of Western civilization?*
*Mahatma Gandhi: I think it would be a very good idea*

## THE SCALE OF THE PROBLEM

### Housing stock

Shelter, along with water, food, warmth and hygienic waste disposal, is a necessity of physical existence, especially in the British climate. A homeless person in Calcutta is better off than a homeless person in London since the weather is less cold. Decent accommodation must be seen as a basic human right in any state that claims to be civilized.

Housing is a very well-researched topic in the UK. Two facts emerge in clear focus from all the research: first, there is a gap of about 100 000 units between the need for and the supply of affordable, decent, rented accommodation; and, second, there is a clear link between inadequate housing and poor health.

In 1992 there were 23 878 000 units of accommodation in the UK. Table 4.1 gives the breakdown of ownership.

**Table 4.1**  Type of accommodation in the UK, 1992

| | | |
|---|---|---|
| Owner-occupied | 15 792 000 | 66.1% |
| Private rented | 2 280 000 | 9.5% |
| Rented from a housing association | 816 000 | 3.4% |
| Rented from new towns, local authorities | 4 990 000 | 20.9% |

[b] This chapter is deeply indebted to the report on the Standing Conference on Public Health (1994) *Housing, Homelessness and Health*. Nuffield Provincial Hospitals Trust. Detailed references are to be found in that chapter.

Of this housing stock, 1 498 000 houses in England (7.4%) were judged to be 'unfit for human habitation' in the official English House Conditions Survey (EHCS) 1991.[1] 95 000 were unfit in Scotland. Unfitness in England means that the house does not meet one or more of the following criteria:

- structurally stable
- free from serious disrepair
- free from health-threatening dampness
- adequate light, heat and ventilation
- adequate piped drinking water
- adequate cooking facilities
- suitably located WC for the occupants' exclusive use
- bath or shower and washing facilities with hot and cold water
- effective drains.

Criteria in Scotland are broadly similar. From these figures, at least 6.7% of the UK housing stock is unfit for human habitation. This is an underestimate because unfit houses in Wales and Northern Ireland have not been included.

Privately owned property and pre-1919 houses are the most likely to be unfit. About one-third of private houses are unfit, and one in five tenants is in a poor situation.

Of the 1 498 000 unfit houses in England, 145 000 (9.7%) stand vacant. In 1992, 142 000 households in England were accepted by councils as officially homeless. There is therefore at least one vacant (unfit) house for every homeless family. Vacant fit houses could be added to this number. Although the location of the homeless does not necessarily match the location of the empty dwellings in every case, this figure does give an indication of the extent to which the housing shortage is a matter of poor distribution, of failure to match existing housing resources (once brought into a usable state) to need.

## Repair costs

The cost of repairing each of the worst 50% of the unfit houses was estimated by the EHCS at £8620, and the average repair cost at between £1130 and £2100 per dwelling, or £3.06 billion overall.[1] Other estimates consider this estimate to be very low and consider £8400 per unit or £12.6 billion overall to be a more realistic figure.

These are large sums when seen as items of expenditure – equivalent to four years' spending on the running costs of the pointless Trident nuclear strikeforce – but, on the other hand, the cost of refurbishing housing can be seen as a very favourable investment. If repairs are not carried out, the fabric of the house deteriorates until the unit is irrevocably lost. If the house is in a terrace, its deterioration may bring others down with it. Thus, £8400 can be seen as a means of preventing the loss of a house, which is the equivalent of producing a house, and as such is an extremely cost-effective investment compared with the £40 000 average cost of building a new unit. In the process of repairing the houses, work is generated, which saves the country the costs of unemployment. Illness caused by poor housing is estimated to cost the NHS £2 billion per year, so that after six years the programme of repair would have paid for itself in terms of health finance alone. Good housing will also make savings in the budgets for temporary accommodation, social services, police, court and prison. Therefore a programme of housing refurbishment must be seen by wise government as an opportunity rather than a liability. In 1995 the Centre for Urban and Regional Research at the University of Sussex carried out a detailed study of these costings.

# Homelessness

The cause of homelessness is simple; not enough low-cost rented accommodation ('social housing') is being provided. During the 1970s 111 000 new houses were started per year; in the 1980s this was cut by more than two-thirds, to 40 000 per year. In 1992:

- 380 000 households made applications to local authorities to be rehoused
- 237 110 (62%) of these applications were rejected as falling outside of the statutory definition of homelessness, so that
- 142 890 households were accepted as homeless by the councils. Of these households
- 62 740 were in temporary accommodation waiting to be rehoused.

There is a very definite upward trend in these figures: for every single household in temporary accommodation in 1980, there were 13 in 1992. The government claims a slight drop in 1993 from 63 070 to 54 010, but this was due to a stricter interpretation of the conditions of acceptance rather than any improvement in the real situation. We cannot escape the conclusion that over the last 15 years the UK has been inexorably sliding away from a state of civilization.

Homelessness is acute in London (69% of English households in temporary accommodation in 1992 were in London) and other great cities, but is by no means restricted to them: rural homelessness tripled between 1988 and 1992. In Scotland between 1982 and 1993, homelessness increased in general by 75%, in rural areas by 95% and in remote areas by 150%. Homelessness has increased more in women (who constitute 70% of officially homeless adults), children (who outnumber adults by 2:1), ethnic minority groups (40–50% of the officially homeless population) and physically disabled people.

# Statutory homelessness

Statutory homelessness is defined under Part III of the 1985 Housing Act as the state of those people in priority need, not intentionally homeless, and with a connection with the local council to which they are applying. Local authorities have a duty to supply permanent housing for this group, and to supply temporary accommodation until housing becomes available. The UK has the second highest levels of homelessness in Europe, and Germany, the UK and France are well ahead of the field in this discreditable respect.

Temporary accommodation means one of the following.

1  *Bed and breakfast*, i.e. houses that have been divided up for the purpose of profiting from council-backed lodgers. (The term is not to be confused with spotlessly clean seaside holiday accommodation, with huge mixed grills provided by cheery landladies.) Since 1991, the numbers in bed and breakfast have begun to fall: in 1994 they had fallen to a third of the 1991 level.
2  *Short-life housing.* This is housing which may be due for demolition within a matter of months, perhaps to make way for a redevelopment scheme.
3  *Hostels.* These are large houses that have been divided up into living units for homeless families. Conditions for quieter families may be made intolerable by the behaviour of noisy neighbours. In at least one hostel, the fire alarms were frequently set off by uncontrolled children so that neighbouring families were subjected to noise stress, and there was a risk that in the not unlikely event of a real fire the fire brigade would not be alerted.
4  *Refuges.* These are specialized hostels, generally to enable women to escape partners who are physically or mentally battering them, and usually provided by campaigning organizations, with local authority support.
5  *Private sector leasing (PSL).* This is the best of available options, available since 1990 when the government made a subsidy available to councils for this purpose. The local authority leases privately owned housing which would otherwise stand empty, partly because of the depressed housing market, and puts it to good use.

For the families involved, life in temporary accommodation means in practical terms:

● frequent moves from place to place. This cause a sense of insecurity for adults and children alike, and disrupts caring services from GPs, health visitors and social workers if it happens that they move to a different administrative area in 'out-of-borough placements'. The average number of moves is three, but 20% of homeless people have to move four times.[2] Half of the moves are at very short notice – less than six days
● overcrowding
● lack of basic amenities
● poor-condition housing
● for those in bed and breakfast, a ten-fold increase in risk of dying in a fire owing to lack of fire escapes and cluttered escape routes
● often being located in expensive areas where shops and amenities are beyond the price range of the family, and where they feel socially isolated

- loss of control over their lives
- a long and uncertain wait for permanent accommodation. The length of wait is rising. In 1987, the average was 33 weeks; in 1991 47 weeks. Larger families tend to stay in temporary accommodation for a longer time than smaller families, since large council houses are not as common as smaller units. Some families of six people in Tower Hamlets have waited in 'temporary accommodation' for ten years.
- the Housing Benefit trap applies to some people who ask for council help, are placed temporarily in bed and breakfast, and finally refused help. Some choose to stay on in bed and breakfast (rather than go out into the street or back to overcrowded relatives who cannot put them up any more) but in order to be able to afford it they give up work in order to qualify for Housing Benefit. This Benefit is paid in arrears, so that they are unable to afford the deposit necessary for private rented accommodation. They are therefore doubly trapped in unemployment and temporary accommodation
- out-of-borough placement may occur if a council discovers that accommodation in a nearby council area is cheaper than accommodation in the home district. Homeless families are therefore transferred to the care of the neighbouring borough, to the financial advantage of the taxpayer, but to the disadvantage of the transferred family, who have to start again with new GPs, health visitors and social workers.

All of these conditions contribute to health problems for families in temporary accommodation. These problems will be detailed below.

## Unofficial homelessness

Many people live with another household. Consider, for example, a young married couple living with parents/in-laws who would far rather live on their own but cannot afford a private rent. They will not be accepted by their local council as homeless unless their parents/in-laws physically throw them out on to the pavement, together with their belongings. In 1991 it was estimated that 1 200 000 households were in this 'concealed homelessness' position in England – a figure more than eight times the figure of 142 000 officially accepted as homeless in 1992.[3]

### Single homeless

Single homelessness accounts for 21% of the total cases of homelessness in London – about 130 000 souls. Case numbers are growing, especially among young girls. It is thought that the increase is the result of changes in the benefits system which make it impossible for young people to afford rent. Forty per cent of roofless young women become homeless in an effort to escape sexual abuse.

Some of these single homeless, unable to find room in a squat, hostel or a friend's floor, end up sleeping rough – the 'roofless'. Numbers of rough sleepers are hard to estimate, and official 1991 census figures of 2703 are almost certainly an underestimate. Shelter's estimate is 2000–3000 in London and 5000 in the rest of the country.

Homeless, or more accurately 'roofless', young people are at risk of exploitation, prostitution, drug and alcohol addiction, crime, tuberculosis and HIV infection.

## Mentally ill homeless

People with mental illnesses on the streets are noticeable, and it is widely supposed that they are the result of the discharge of inmates of psychiatric hospitals to the 'community'. Two reports,[4,5] have suggested that this is not the case, and that the mentally ill seen on the street have never been in contact with the psychiatric services. In view of the difficulty of accurately surveying street people, and the direct anecdotal evidence of psychiatric workers who have seen their ex-patients on the street, it remains to be seen if the 'community' psychiatry initiative has been completely successful.

## Access to health care

The delivery of health care to homeless people raises special problems. Often penniless, they cannot afford public transport fares, and may be too far from the GP surgery to walk, especially if they have been given an out-of-borough placement. Appointment times are often missed, owing to the vagaries of the street life; finding food or a place to sleep may take priority at the set time, or the passing of time may simply not register. Their appearance, attitudes and odour may cause difficulties in communication with receptionists and doctors, who may often see them as problem patients. A GP in Bedford who supplies medical care to six hostels for the homeless writing in *GP Magazine* has calculated that he actually makes a loss out of the service he provides to these patients. He commented, 'The ethics of the market have taken over the ethics of care. People who have maximum need get minimum care'. For all of these reasons, it is desirable that health authorities should set up special services dedicated to the needs of the homeless.

## The health problems of the unofficial homeless

These begin with a high mortality rate.[6] Eighty-six homeless people died in the year to August 1991, with an average age of 47 years and a total mortality rate 2.8 times higher than expected. Most were men, and nearly one in four deaths was due to suicide. Assault was the most common cause of death, followed by suicide, accident, pneumonia and hypothermia.[7]

Studies of morbidity (illness) are impeded by the difficulty of keeping tabs on the roofless. Their GP consultation rates are not increased, but they have more skin and cardiovascular problems.[8]

# HEALTH OF THE OFFICIALLY HOMELESS

## Temporary accommodation

The health of homeless families in temporary accommodation has been extensively studied, and clear evidence exists that homelessness is associated with ill-health, not all of which can be assumed to exist before the family became homeless.[9,10]

Facilities for cooking, washing, excretion and escape in event of fire for those in temporary accommodation are inadequate, as has been set out above, and access to health care and social workers may be more difficult.

Pregnant women in temporary accommodation have twice as many medical problems with their pregnancy as adequately housed women. Women who become homeless during pregnancy are three times more likely to be admitted to hospital during the pregnancy, and are more likely to have a Caesarean section and anaemia than women who become homeless after the birth.

Babies born to homeless women are more likely to be premature or under-weight (25% have low birthweight compared with 10% overall), and to have difficulty in breathing.[11]

Children in temporary accommodation are prone to behavioural disturbance, including developmental delay, aggression, poor sleep and bedwetting.[12,13]

Mental health problems include increased smoking and drinking, depression, suicide attempts and relationship problems. Families become isolated from relatives and friends, and self-esteem disappears.

Physical health deteriorates in temporary accommodation, with increases measured in lung tuberculosis, rheumatic aches and skin, neurological and respiratory diseases.[14,15]

# HEALTH OF THE UNOFFICIALLY HOMELESS

About one in three roofless people, rough sleepers and hostel dwellers abuses alcohol.[16] The effects of heavy drinking together with inadequate nutrition (alcohol inhibits absorption of fat-soluble vitamins) mean that complications of alcoholism are commonplace, including duodenal ulcers, peripheral neuritis (malfunction of nerves to the limbs), weak legs, blackouts and injuries. Alcohol-induced aggression can lead to injuries, arrest and being barred from helping agencies. Drug abuse was only found in 10% of this study group.[16]

As with those in temporary accommodation, musculoskeletal, skin and respiratory disorders are common. Half have chronic (longstanding) physical diseases, and a fifth have more than one disease. Tuberculosis is an important disease of rough sleepers, especially as, *faute de mieux*, they must spit on the street, where the bacillus dries and rises into the air ready to infect the next undernourished person who comes along. In the USA, rough sleepers are a reservoir of tuberculosis bacilli that are resistant to common antibacterial agents.

Psychiatric disorder is common among the roofless. Half of the residents at one hostel were sufficiently psychiatrically disabled to qualify for admission to a hospital, yet were being managed without medication in the community by untrained staff.[17] Other studies give figures for major psychiatric illness of between 20 and 80%.[18]

Imprisonment is often the result of subsistence stealing (for food or milk) or mentally disordered behaviour. Nearly two-thirds of men remanded to Winchester prison for psychiatric reports between 1979 and 1983 were homeless at the time of their arrest.[19] Prison is often an attractive option, since it offers shelter, warmth, food and medical care. The cost of this kind of imprisonment is outside of the scope of this book, yet should be included in any overall costing of a strategic approach to Britain's housing problems.

Temporary accommodation and rough sleeping are associated with significant health problems. Reverse causality – the fact that poor mental and physical health will tend to produce 'downward social mobility' – undoubtedly plays a small part in the observed ill-health, but the mental stresses and physical conditions of homelessness must be considered to be responsible for causing the overwhelming majority of the problems.

Although the health problems of the homeless are undertreated, those that are treated tend to be dealt with by hospitals rather than in primary care, and this is an inefficient way of delivering health care. In the case of at least one disease – tuberculosis – this undertreatment cannot be seen as a case for self-congratulation by administrators keen on saving money, since one case not treated today may mean ten cases to be treated in five years' time.

# HEALTH IMPACT OF POOR HOUSING

## Mortality and morbidity rates

People who own their own homes live longer than those who live in rented accommodation. Child mortality is higher in those living in rented council houses (it is also associated with overcrowding, lack of amenities, and male unemployment).[20] The findings for illness (morbidity) rates are similar, with more health problems being reported from people in rented accommodation. The differences are more marked among young women.

It is impossible to say from these figures alone whether, and to what extent, the association is likely to be due to the general effects of deprivation, of which poor home conditions is one factor.

# Low indoor temperature

People die in winter. Each winter about 40 000 more people die in the UK than in the previous summer months (Table 4.2). In European countries with colder winters but homes that are better insulated and heated, there are fewer excess winter deaths. The colder the UK winter, the more people die: about 8000 extra deaths for each degree Celsius that the temperature falls below the average.[21] These deaths are over and above the average expected deaths for that year; after a peak of deaths, there is no fall in reported deaths, which is what we would expect if the cold had only brought forward a fated demise.

Heart disease, respiratory disease and stroke are the main causes of death associated with cold.[22,23] There is evidence that blood pressure rises in the elderly when exposed to cold.

Only a small percentage of cold-related deaths are caused by hypothermia – about 168 deaths each winter.

Unemployed, chronic sick and elderly people have to stay at home all day, often in an inactive state. This means that their fuel bills will increase. They will tend to save money by heating only one room, which leads to stress from the difference in temperature as they move from room to room. The temperature differential also causes condensation.

Condensation occurs when air containing water vapour comes in contact with a surface sufficiently cold to reduce the air temperature below dew point. Within a house it occurs through an imbalance between the provision of heating, the levels of insulation and the rate of ventilation.

Condensation is increased by:

- reducing the heating, which gives higher levels of relative humidity together with colder surfaces
- lack of insulation if this results in lower temperatures in the house
- insufficient ventilation to remove damp air from the house. Excessive ventilation causes cold air and more condensation.

Moulds dislike the salty moisture associated with rising damp, and prefer the pure moisture of condensation. Proliferation of moulds leads in turn to allergic disease

**Table 4.2** Temperature and health risk

| Temperature (°C) | |
| --- | --- |
| 21 | Recommended temperature for elderly |
| 18 | Comfort level for most people |
| 16 | Respiratory problems increase |
| 13 | Standard for kitchens |
| 12 | Increased risk of heart disease/stroke |
| 5 | Risk of hypothermia |

in the airways. Paraffin and gas heaters, which are more likely to be used by people on low incomes, also lead to increased condensation. Badly burning gas heaters also contribute to indoor air pollution.

Low-cost homes are hard to heat. Concrete has a high thermal mass, absorbing much heat before the room feels warm. Concrete beams and metal wall ties act as cold bridges, conducting heat out of the living space. Doors and windows in cheap pre-fabricated houses and flats are often ill-fitting, causing heat loss through draughts.

Poor households spend twice as much on heating as a proportion of their income as the better off (11% as opposed to 5.4%).

To get a rough feel for the impact of cold housing on the NHS, let us assume that, of the 8000 deaths associated with a drop of 1°C, half occur in hospital, and that for each person that dies five are taken to hospital and survive. Let us also assume that one stay in hospital costs £1000.

Total number of cold-affected cases = 5 × 8000 = 40 000 + 8000 = 48 000.
Number of hospital admissions = 48 000 − 4000 (who die at home) = 44 000.
Cost of hospital admissions resulting from a 1°C drop in temperature =
44 000 × £1000 = £44 000 000 for each degree Celsius drop in temperature.
For a 5°C drop in temperature, the cost is £220 million.

## The treatment of fuel poverty

Warmth is a fundamental prerequisite for life, and should be seen as a basic human right, but if bleeding-heart considerations of human rights cut no ice, even hard-headed financial considerations drive us to the same conclusion. If we were to rectify the poorly insulated state of Britain's homes it would result in significant savings for the NHS – more than £800 million in Dr Boardman's estimation.[24] It would also lead to significant long-term savings to the fabric of the country's housing stock, as cold, damp housing deteriorates more rapidly. A total of 500 000 job–years of work would be created in the act of insulating all of Britain's houses to European standards.

Instead, because of a policy decision taken in February 1988 to target home insulation grants only to applicants on low incomes, insulation installations plummeted. Woodspring District Council's figures (Table 4.3) show a 20-fold drop in insulation grants following this decision (personal communication). It cannot be assumed that those who would have benefited 'went private' for their insulation needs since, at a domestic level, payback considerations of smaller fuel bills in the future are not effective. Faced with large capital bills for insulation, most households on medium incomes will simply abandon the idea of insulating their property.

**Table 4.3**  Woodspring District Council insulation applications approved

| 1986–87 | 1987–88 | 1988–89 | 1989–90 |
|---------|---------|---------|---------|
| 1486    | 969     | 51      | 28      |

## The Energy Conservation Bill

The Energy Conservation Bill (ECB) was drawn up by the Green Party's campaign manager, Ron Bailey, in alliance with the Association for Conservation of Energy and other interested organizations. It was presented to Parliament by the Plaid/Green MP Cynog Dafis with backing from Conservative, Liberal Democrat and Labour MPs. An intensive lobbying campaign followed, spearheaded by the Green Party, and a majority of MP's support for the Bill was obtained. Alan Beith MP, the Liberal Democrat deputy leader won the Private Members' ballot, a kind of Parliamentary lottery, and chose to present the ECB. Surprisingly, over 70 Tory MPs who had signed the motion 'welcoming' the Bill trooped into the lobby to support the government motion to 'deplore' it. Robert Jones MP, a Conservative Chair of the Environment Select Committee wrote 'I am very glad to support the ECB. It is long overdue. I shall urge the government to support it. I will sponsor the Bill.' At the time of the vote, he wrote 'Frankly we have much more important practical things to get on with. I deplore the Bill.'

Tenaciously, Ron Bailey and the Green Party continued the pressure, and it reappeared as the Energy Conservation and Warmer Homes Bill. At the next Private Members' ballot, Diana Maddocks, another Liberal Democrat MP, won the right to present a Bill, and again took the opportunity to present the Energy Conservation Bill. This time, mindful of the political damage they had sustained when they had talked it out, the government accepted the Bill. Under the Energy Conservation Act, local authorities are obliged to conduct an energy survey of local properties and draw up plans to improve energy conservation measures, together with estimates for financial costs and the resultant saving of carbon dioxide. There will be a statement of the council's policy for taking into account the 'personal circumstances' (poverty, age, disability etc.) of households surveyed. The Secretary of State must set times for reports and reviews to come back, and has indicated that he will seek a 30% reduction initially. He must assist councils with resourcing the Act, and must report back to Parliament on progress.

The Energy Conservation Bill offsets the increased cost due to the introduction of VAT on fuel to the lower paid by reducing the amount of fuel which we need to use. The cost-effectiveness of the measure is increased by lower housing maintenance costs estimated at £100–£500 per annum per dwelling due to less dampness in housing.

The conclusion is that concerted effort to improve Britain's poorly insulated homes would result in significant savings for the NHS. It would also lead to significant long-term savings to the fabric of the country's housing stock, as cold, damp housing deteriorates more rapidly. 500 000 job–years of work would be created in the act of insulating all of Britain's houses to European standards.

## Solving the problem: the Glasgow Heatwise experience

In 1989 Glasgow City Council made a survey of their housing stock and found that, in a city of 290 000 dwellings, 36% were affected by one of either dampness, condensation or mould growth. Four per cent of the stock was affected by all three.[25]

In response to this finding, Heatwise Glasgow's Jobs and Energy Project began work in the Easterhouse estate, where the least energy-efficient houses were to be found: some of the walls of the houses in the estate lost heat three to five times as fast as walls built to current standards. An energy audit of 30 dwellings concluded that the occupants should be spending up to four times as much as the Scottish average on domestic heating to bring their room temperature up to a reasonable level. However, a survey of actual expenditure showed that, although they were spending more than the average, and much more than the official allowance in the welfare benefit calculations for fuel consumption, they were still underheating their homes, and so incurring problems of damp, cold and mould.

Four homes were then chosen for improvements aimed to meet or surpass the thermal standards of the Scottish Building Regulations. Work was carried out using local labour (which had another benefit of improving local incomes) to insulate the properties with:

- wall cavity and external cladding
- double-glazed UPVC windows to replace the original ill-fitting windows
- at least 150 mm of insulation in the loft space
- whole-house heating that also provided hot water
- draughtproofing of doors
- ventilation improvements
- enclosed balcony spaces.

The cost for this was £5000 per unit with a payback time of seven years measured by 'before and after' costs of heating the units to a reasonable standard. The occupants gained warmer homes for lower fuel expenditure (falling from £20 per week to £2 per week to bring the house up to the same heating standard), the local economy benefited from the work created, and the local medical services should have benefited from a reduction in consultations for illness by those living in the improved houses. The whole community and the next generation will benefit from the longer useful life of the buildings protected by warmer, drier internal conditions.

## Dampness and mould

The English House Condition Survey 1991 found that dampness was present in 10% of occupied public sector houses and 24% of occupied private houses.

Cold and dampness almost always coexist, and each multiplies the adverse health effects of the other.

House dust mites, fungi, pathogenic (disease producing) bacteria and viruses all thrive in damp houses. Fungi are particularly fond of the kind of damp produced by condensation. *Alternaria, Cladosporium, Penicillium* and *Aspergillus* are the domestic fungi most commonly involved with allergic reactions.

Damp houses are associated with respiratory disease, especially wheezing in children,[26,27] and there is a known association between indoor moulds and asthma,[28] rhinitis[29] (a hayfever-like condition that occurs throughout the year) and alveolitis[30] (a serious condition in which the air sacs of the lungs become progressively ineffective, resulting in severe shortness of breath).

In Edinburgh, the incidence of wheeze and chesty cough among children who slept in damp rooms was found to be 22% – twice that of children who slept in dry rooms.[31] However, although there was a strong correlation between visible mould and the parents' report that their children wheezed, there was no correlation between reports of mould and objective measurements of bronchial function. The inference from this is that reporting bias may be affecting the results, so that parents who saw mould on the walls were more likely to report that their children were wheezing. Two explanations are possible for this: either the wheeze report was exaggerated in the hope of getting something done about the mould, or the parents in the damp houses actually perceived their children to be less healthy. In so far as this perception is operating, it is still an important measure of lack of well-being, since part of a person's total health consists in a subjective sense of well-being.

In order to overcome the problem of self-reporting of damp, environmental health officers surveyed damp and mould independently.[32,33] It was found that dampness was associated with respiratory allergy and infection (sore throat, coughing) in children, and also aches and pains. No correlation with adult illness was found. Social class, unemployment, overcrowding, smoking, cooking, pets, number of children in the home and family income were all excluded as possible confounding factors.

A confirmatory study showed associations between dampness/mould and respiratory symptoms, diarrhoea, vomiting and poor general health.[34] Further confirmation for the connection between mould and ill-health comes from a very large study in Canada.[35]

Laboratory studies show that moulds can affect health in three ways: through allergy, infection and the effects of their mycotoxins. The illness that they cause can vary from mild cold-like symptoms, through influenza-like aches and weakness, to severe chronic breathlessness.

Damp and mould appear to be strongly associated with depression. No mechanisms are known to account for this in physical terms, so it must be supposed that the cause is the unpleasant look and feel of the place.

The conclusion, beyond all reasonable doubt, is that cold, damp houses cause mould growth, and moulds cause illness. Action to produce warmer, drier houses will save the NHS money and will lead to a healthier, more productive population. As a side-effect of this action, structural housing problems of corrosion, decay and electrical wiring faults (including fires caused by these faults) will be reduced.

## Overheating

Generally, the hotter the indoor air, the lower the humidity, that is the drier the air. Table 4.4 shows the effects of humidity.

There is some evidence that at low levels of humidity the resistance of the mucous membranes to infection is lowered, and therefore the chances of getting colds and viruses are increased.[36,37] More research is needed on this topic.

## Overcrowding

The transmission of infectious diseases occurs more readily in overcrowded living space. It has been known for many years that tuberculosis and dysentery are rife in overcrowded slums. *Helicobacter pylori*, which has recently been found guilty of causing gastric ulcers and possibly gastric carcinoma, is another bacterium the spread of which is helped by overcrowding, and areas with high gastric carcinoma are also those which have had high levels of overcrowding in the past.[38] Peptic ulcers in females are associated with current overcrowding.

It is difficult to separate out the effects of overcrowding from other factors such as deprivation and smoking when interpreting research results, but some non-infective conditions do seem to be associated with overcrowding:

- accidental and violent deaths including suicide
- heart attack and stroke, especially in males
- cancer of cervix and lung
- chronic bronchitis, asthma and emphysema; regardless of smoking habits.[39]

The effects of overcrowding in children carry through into adult life, being manifested as an increased risk of heart attacks, chronic bronchitis and emphysema. An

**Table 4.4**   Effects of humidity

| Relative humidity level | |
| --- | --- |
| Relative humidity level (%) | Effect |
| 70 | Damp air<br>Probability of mould growth increased<br>Air-borne pathogens (disease-causing bacteria) survive longer |
| 40 | Dry air<br>Electric shocks generated by carpets<br>House dust mite population falls |
| 30 | Severe electric shocks from carpets<br>Mucous membranes (eyes, nose, throat) become dry and irritated<br>Drying and cracking of skin and nails |

adult who suffered overcrowding as an infant is liable to have chronic cough and poor lung function, possibly as a result of the repeated respiratory infections that are a feature of sharing space with many others. In addition, gastric (stomach) ulceration in adults is associated with overcrowding as a child.

Mental health is also affected by overcrowding, with women at home with small children in poor conditions particularly likely to be affected.[40] Women appear to suffer more in conditions of congestion, that is when demands are made by many people on the use of one particular space. This takes away individuals' sense of control of their space and therefore of their life. This recalls the findings of Marmot's lower rank civil servants[41] and of Newman's theories of 'defensible space' – space that is under personal control.[42] On the other hand, stress effects due to overcrowding were not much in evidence in one study of the severely overcrowded conditions in Hong Kong,[43] although these findings have been contradicted by other research.

Houses in multiple occupation (HMO) is a term that covers houses that have been converted into flats, student lodgings, hostels and the bed and breakfast facilities used by local authorities to house those who are deemed to be homeless. Often families have to share facilities for washing, cooking, food storage and excretion. Because nobody has overall responsibility for the common areas, hygiene in these areas is usually poor. Infectious diseases, especially childhood diarrhoeas, are common in HMOs.[44] Conditions are usually overcrowded, and passageways are often used to store possessions. Fire is a major hazard; it is more likely to break out, and when that happens there are many people to be evacuated, often through ill-designed and obstructed exit points.

## Recommendation

That the government should act on the advice of the Institute of Environmental Health Officers (IEHO) to introduce national codes of practice and mandatory inspection and licensing of HMOs.

# Neighbour noise

Complaints of neighbour noise to local council environmental health departments have risen 20-fold over the last 20 years, and are still rising at a rate of about 10% per year. One study showed that 56% of people are annoyed by noise at home. Scotland is an exception, with static complaint levels. It is thought that the reasons for this are that (a) Scottish houses are built to better standards than English houses and (b) it is the police rather than environmental health officers, who are the agents who deal with noise complaints. It is not clear whether the effect of this situation is to make people as quiet as mice in their houses or whether people simply do not complain since the consequence of grassing-up the neighbours to the police is far more severe than the consequence of putting up with a little noise.

The most frequent source of noise annoyance is the neighbours, if their children, dogs and car alarms are included. Next comes general road traffic noise, followed by motorcycles, although complaints about motorcycles have fallen significantly since 1985 because of new noise emission standards. Aircraft noise is next in terms of the annoyance it causes, followed by noise from industry, places of entertainment, schools and trains.

Studies have shown that noise generated by people is more annoying than impersonal noise made by traffic, railways and industry. Being able to hear the neighbours implies that the neighbours can also hear you; this creates a sense of lack of privacy, and loss of privacy is a source of stress.

Noise problems are worse in non-traditionally constructed houses since the thin slab blocks transmit sound. More than half of the walls of newly completed houses fail to meet the Building Research Establishment's recommended noise transmission standards. It seems that about half of the problem arises from poor structural materials and half from inconsiderate behaviour or poor planning. For instance, domestic noise complaints will be worse in areas where young children are housed alongside elderly people.

# Accidents

Forty per cent of all fatal accidents occur in the home. Five thousand people lost their lives in domestic accidents in 1991 – roughly the same number as died in road traffic accidents. The cost of domestic accidents to the NHS in England and Wales is about £300 million a year.[45] The number of accidents is not surprising as we spend 75–94% of our time in the home.

Domestic accidents are the commonest cause of death in children aged over 12 months;[46] they account for a third of all childhood deaths and one quarter of all deaths between the age of ten and 14 years. About 50% of accidents to children at home are associated with bad design of accommodation.

Falls account for 60% of home accidents and fire for 15%. People in lower social classes and income brackets tend to have more accidents and fires. The class gradient for childhood deaths by accident is steeper (that is more positively related) than for any other cause of death in children.[47]

Older people in the early stages of dementia living alone are at risk of explosion and fire from switching the gas on and forgetting to light it. Gas detector alarms already exist, and it would be a small step to link these detectors to the gas-off switch.

The Child Accident Prevention Trust has produced guidelines to make homes safer. It recommends that new houses should be planned with:

● L-shaped flights of stairs
● no doors or windows opening on to stairs
● through routes in kitchens that avoid the cooker.

In addition, it suggests that existing homes could be made safer by:

- improving lighting of stairwells
- introducing handrails with an all-round grab
- removing cupboards above the cooker
- laying non-slip floors in the kitchen
- installing safety glazing for shower screens, glass doors and French windows.

Glass breakages account for approximately 50% of lacerations to children – some 400 000 events needing emergency treatment per year. Legislation covering safety glass at the moment is obscure. The government should change the building regulations to ensure that all low-level door panels (the most likely to be involved in a falling accident) are made from toughened safety glass.

Fire accounts for 15% of domestic accidents, and approximately 700 deaths per year. The incidence is associated with unemployment, low socioeconomic status and living in rented property.[48] Forty-three per cent of fire deaths occur in those over 60 years of age.

Carbon monoxide poisoning accounts for 100 deaths per year, mainly from fumes from badly installed or badly maintained appliances. Low-grade carbon monoxide poisoning may cause Parkinson's disease.

## Insecurity

Homes are about security. Security is an emotional tie to any place associated with love and a sense of identity, and the emotion is especially poignant for children. Fear of eviction may cause depression in some people. Personal historic attachments can be very strong, and can overcome a multitude of physical defects in the accommodation. Often older people will cling to their own home even though it is clear to themselves and all around that they are unable to cope on their own and are at risk of falls, fire and gassing. Whereas in theory home ownership has the advantage of freeing people from the insecurity of the tenant relationship, in practice the result for some has been a transition from secure council tenancy to owner-occupier status, to unemployment, to eviction and temporary accommodation, which is the ultimate in home insecurity.

Eviction for inability to meet mortgage repayments is often an irrational process the only effect of which is to punish the occupier. In some cases the mortgage company throws one family on to the tender mercies of the local authority's homelessness programme, and the house stands empty until sold to another family who stay there until their breadwinner likewise is made redundant. Any occupier who runs into difficulty should be able to convert flexibly to a part-mortgage, part-rent scheme, such as that increasingly being used for 'first rung' buyers.

Harassment by unscrupulous landlords and/or racists is a common source of insecurity. Technology could be used to reduce this by placing an alarm call system (which is often supplied to the frail elderly) to people who feel they are being harassed.

## Flats

Many commentators, viewing the high-rise flats of the 1950s and 1960s, instinctively condemned them as hostile environments. A visitor finds cramped, cold, noisy, impersonal, vandalized and dirty private and public spaces. Residents and visitors develop a fear of attack in dark alleys. The lack of play areas gives rise to a sense of imprisonment for children and their carers. Broken lifts and vandalized, uriniferous stairs compound the sense of isolation. Rubbish accumulates in public spaces, as nobody has responsibility for cleaning it up.

These observations and feelings were dismissed by architects and experts responsible for the flats for two decades until sufficient undeniable evidence accumulated to show that this form of development was a mistake. Ronan Point, in London, a corner of which physically collapsed in 1968, contributed to the loss of faith in the high rise even on the part of their advocates. Meanwhile, the high-rise flat culture has spread throughout the world.

Morbidity (poor health) is 50% higher among those living in flats than among those living in houses.[49] People living in flats have been found to have more symptoms of mental ill-health than those in houses, and the effect is more marked the higher the block.[50] A survey of the Divis flats in Belfast showed that 70% of households had at least one member who showed signs of depression or mental stress. Factors associated with this were the military presence, violence, poor housing, poverty and unemployment.

Neighbour noise is worse in flats, partly because of poor construction and partly because neighbours are not just to either side of the home, but also above and below.

The solution to the problem of flat living does not necessarily involve physically destroying them and rebuilding new accommodation. If a sense of community and common purpose is present among the residents of the flats, much can be done to improve the problems. The critical aim should be to develop a sense of common ownership and common responsibility for the building and the surrounding area.

In one instance a sick elderly lady in a high-rise flat in Hartcliffe, Bristol, was part of a small spontaneous community of ladies who shared a common landing. In contrast to the bare concrete floor of other landings, this common space was carpeted ('We got the punks downstairs to fetch it up for us out of the skip'). They formed a mutually supportive group of five or six friends, and the atmosphere was positive and entirely different from that in the typical apartment.

The history of the Hermes and Chantry Points, two 21-storey blocks on the Elgin estate in Westminster, is an example of the power of a community in improving its situation, although it ended in failure. In 1985 Westminster City Council decided to sell the flats to the highest bidder. The tenants objected to their homes being sold

(Figure 4.1), and for three years they frustrated the council's plans. They formed a company, and forced Westminster, under the provisions of the 1988 Housing Act, to give them freehold to the estates and all the money they needed to carry out long overdue repairs. After some three years of living in what was described as a 'vertical village', it was discovered that asbestos was leaking into the living space and the flats had to be abandoned. Pete Stockwell (personal communication), one of the group of activists in the community, wrote:

> For those of us who lived in Hermes and Chantry, those years were a real treat. The flats were well designed, light poured in through windows reminiscent of a cross channel ferry, and the view from the upper floor was fantastic. More importantly, we proved that tower block living doesn't have to be a J G Ballard nightmare. There was a tremendous sense of community...between all residents... At the same time, of course, it's important to underline the fact that a sense of community alone does not eradicate poverty, damp or cockroaches.

Concierges can help to develop a sense of common ownership in flats. By making one person responsible for the tidiness, cleanliness and general well-being of the flats, a job is created, and a sense of responsibility is introduced not just in the concierge but, by his or her efforts, in the community at large.

On the other hand, sometimes conditions in flats are so unacceptable that it is necessary to demolish and rebuild them. The Divis flats in Belfast were the subject of a long campaign on the part of the residents to get themselves rehoused. For

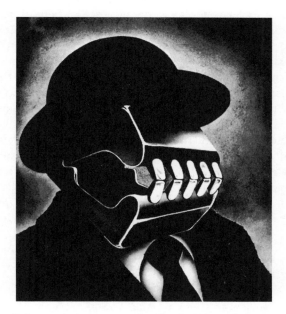

**Figure 4.1**  'We are a little worried about our landlord'. Acknowledgement: Walterton and Elgin Action Group. Artist: John Phillips.

years nothing was done by local or national politicians, until local people began to take direct action. When a flat became empty, the community would move in to smash the flat into a totally uninhabitable state. This action was successful where conventional pressure was ineffective.

# COUNTING THE COST OF POOR HOUSING

## NHS costs

The impact of inadequate accommodation on NHS spending has been estimated by looking at a problem that is known to cause a certain amount of illness, multiplying it by the number of people known to be affected by the problem, and then multiplying it by the amount of NHS money required to treat one case of that illness. Using this method, Boardman assessed the cost to the NHS of illness caused by cold housing alone at £800 000 000.[24] Carr-Hill and Coyle[51] apparently surveyed people in poor housing, using a health diary, and found that their use of NHS services was 50% higher than normal. Extrapolating their data to cover the whole population affected by poor housing, they arrived at the conclusion that the NHS was spending £2 billion per year – 6% of the budget – on trying to treat conditions caused by poor housing.

Unfortunately, the Department of Health did not permit the publication of the research paper, and the authors are not able freely to discuss their research methods and findings. Nevertheless, in the absence of better figures, this figure of £2 billion will be used here as the cost to the NHS of poor housing. It is a conservative figure, since it is not thought that the Carr-Hill and Coyle paper covered the very significant extra costs of temporary accommodation and rooflessness.

Two billion pounds is such a huge sum and such a significant part of the health service budget that it might cause even the most hard-nosed politician to take an interest in the matter. Politicians for whom money is an absolute might well be unmoved by the human suffering of families and individuals without physical protection in our cold climate, but the thought of large sums of taxpayers' money being wasted on illnesses that are capable of being prevented might just be enough to motivate them. For others, the motivation would be to bring about a situation where housing is available to all, and therefore for Britain to be qualified to answer to the name of 'civilized'. The question is, how much will it cost to rectify the situation? The next chapter will attempt to answer this question.

# REFERENCES

1   Department of Environment (1993) *English House Conditions Survey 1991.* HMSO, London.

2   Tritter and Edwards (1993) *The experience of homeless families in private sector leased temporary accommodation.* South Bank University, London.

3   Office of Population Censuses and Surveys (1992) *Survey of Sharers 1990.* OPCS, London.

4   Craig T, Hepworth C, Klein O *et al.* (1993) *Homelessness and Mental Health Initiative: Second Report to the Mental Health Foundation.* RDP.

5   North East Thames Regional Health Authority Team for Assessment Psychiatric Services (TAPS) (1990). London.

6   Royal College of Physicians of London (1994) *Homelessness and Ill Health.* Royal College of Physicians, London.

7   Keyes S and Kennedy M (1992) *Sick to Death of Homelessness.* Crisis, London.

8   Bazals J (1993) Health care for the single homeless. In: K Fisher (ed.) *Homelessness, Health Care and Welfare Provision.* Routledge, London.

9   Health Visitor's Association and the BMA (1989) *Homeless families and their health.* Health Visitor's Association and the BMA, London.

10  Conway J (1988) *Prescription for Poor Health: the Crisis for Homeless Families.* London Food Commission, Maternity Alliance, SHAC, Shelter, London.

11  Audit Commission (1986) *Managing the crisis in council housing.* HMSO, London.

12  Lovell B (1986) Health visiting homeless families. *Health Visitor*: **59**; 334–7.

13  Boyer J (1986) Homelessness from a health visitor's point of view. *Health Visitor*: **59**; 342–3.

14  Shanks N and Carroll K (1984) Persistent tuberculosis disease among inmates of common lodging houses. *J Epidemiol Commun Health*: **36**; 130–4.

15  Shanks N (1988) Medical Morbidity of the Homeless. *J Epidemiol Commun Health*: **42**; 183–6.

16  Toon P D, Thomas K and Doherty M (1987) Audit of work at a medical centre for the homeless over one year. *J R Coll Gen Pract*: **37**; 120–2.

17  Marshall M (1989) Collected and neglected: are Oxford hostels for the homeless filling up with disabled psychiatric patients? *BMJ*: **299**; 706–9.

18  James A (1989) Homeless women in London: the hostel perspective. *Health Trends*: **21**; 70–1.

19  Mental Health Foundation (1993) *Diversion, care and justice.* Conference documents, London.

20  Brennan M E and Lancashire R (1978) Association of childhood mortality with housing status and unemployment. *J Epidemiol Commun Health*: **32**; 28–33.

21  Bull G and Morton J (1978) Environment, temperature and death rates. *Age and Ageing*: 7; 210–24.

22    Editorial (1980) Blows from the winter wind. *BMJ*: **i**; 137–8.

23    Bull G and Morton J (1978) Environment, temperature and death rates. *Age and Ageing*: **7**; 210–24.

24    Boardman B (1991) *Fuel Poverty*. Bellhaven Press, London.

25    Sheldrick B and Alembic Research (1994) Paper presented to the NSCA Environmental Protection Conference. Glasgow.

26    Burr M L, St Leger A S, Yarnell J W G (1981) Wheezing, dampness, and coal fires. *Commun Med*: **3**; 205–9.

27    Burr M L, Miskelly F G, Butland B K *et al.* (1989) Environmental factors and symptoms in infants at high risk of allergy. *J Epidemiol Commun Health*: **43**; 125–32.

28    Burr M L, Mullins J, Merrett T G *et al.* (1988) Indoor moulds and asthma. *J R Soc Health*: **108**; 99–101.

29    Solomon W R (1974) Fungus aerosols arising from cold mist vaporisers. *J Allergy*: **54**; 222–8.

30    Fergusson R, Milne L, Crompton G (1984) Penicillium allergic alveolitis: faulty installation of central heating. *Thorax*: **39**; 294–8.

31    Burridge R and Ormandy D (1993) *Unhealthy Housing: Research, Remedies and Reform*. E&FN Spon, London.

32    Martin C J, Platt S D, Hunt S M (1987) Housing conditions and ill health. *BMJ*: **294**; 1125–7.

33    Platt C D, Martin C J, Hunt S M *et al.* (1989) Damp housing, mould growth, and symptomatic health state. *BMJ*: **298**; 1673–8.

34    Hyndman S J (1990) Housing dampness and health among British Bengalis in East London. *Soc Sci Med*: **30**; 131–41.

35    Dales R E, Zwanenburg H, Burnerr R *et al.* (1991) Respiratory health effects of home dampness and moulds among Canadian children. *Am J Epidemiol*: **134**; 196–203.

36    Green G H (1982) Positive and negative effects of building humidification. *Ashrae Trans*: **88**, part 1.

37    Health implications of the level of indoor air humidity (1984) Proceedings of the Conference on Indoor Air, Stockholm.

38    Barker D J P, Coggon D, Osmond C *et al.* (1990) Poor housing in childhood and high rates of stomach cancer in England and Wales. *Br J Cancer*: **61**; 575–8.

39    Kellet J M (1989) Health and Housing. *J Psychosomatic Res*: **33**; 255–68.

40    Brown G W and Harris T (1978) *Social origins of depression*. Tavistock publications, London.

41    Marmot M G, Shipley M J, Rose G (1984) Inequalities in Death – Specific explanations of a general pattern? *Lancet*: **i**; 1003–4.

**42**  Newman D (1972) *Defensible Space: Crime Prevention through Urban Design.* Macmillan, New York.

**43**  Mitchell R E (1971) Some social implications of high density housing. *Am Sociol Rev*: **36**; 18–29.

**44**  Conway J (1988) *Prescription for Poor Health. The Health Crisis for Homeless Families.* London Food Commission, Maternity Alliance, SHAC, Shelter, London.

**45**  Department of Trade and Industry (1989) *Home and Leisure Accident Research. Eleventh annual report accident surveillance system: 1987 data.* DTI, London.

**46**  DHSS (1986) *On the state of the public health for the year 1985.* The Annual Report of the Chief Medical Officer of the DHSS. HMSO, London.

**47**  DHSS (1980) *Report of the Working Group on Inequalities in Health (The Black Report).* DHSS, London.

**48**  Chandler S E, Chapman A, Hollington S J (1984) Fire incidence, housing and social conditions – the urban situation in Britain. *Fire Prev*: **172**; 15–20.

**49**  Fanning D M (1967) Families in flats. *BMJ*: **iv**; 382–6.

**50**  Hannay D R (1981) Mental health and high flats. *J Chroni Dis*: **34**; 431–2.

**51**  Carr-Hill R A, Coyle D, Ivens C (1993) Poor Housing: Poor Health? Unpublished report funded by the Department of the Environment, London.

# 5

# Solutions to the housing crisis

*The strength of a nation is derived from the integrity of its homes*

Confucius

## A DECENT HOME FOR EVERY FAMILY?

When we remember that there are about 380 000 applications per year to be rehoused, 145 000 empty houses in need of refurbishment, 500 000 construction workers drawing Unemployment Benefit and £5.5 billion in district councils' capital receipts budgets, and when we remind ourselves that the bill to the NHS for treating illness caused by inadequate housing is £2 billion per year, the real difficulty lies in understanding why the government does not invest in a major programme of house rehabilitation and building immediately.

Instead, housebuilding is an area of the economy from which the government has been making sustained and deliberate efforts to extricate itself (Table 5.1).

This figure shows how government spending on housing, although substantially unaltered overall, has moved away from building to MITR and housing benefits. Housing subsidy has moved from building production to the demand side.

**Table 5.1** Government expenditure on housebuilding

| Year | Housing (£bn) | MITR (£bn) | Housing Benefit (£bn) |
|------|------|------|------|
| 1979–80 | 13 | 3.3 | |
| 1985–86 | | | 3.1 |
| 1991–92 | 5.8 | 6.1 | |
| 1992–93 | | | 7.3 |

MITR, mortgage interest tax relief.

Housing and construction statistics, quoted in a Catholic Housing Aid Society (CHAS) publication,[1] show that dwelling starts (both local authority and housing association) fell from 91 153 in 1979 to 43 300 in 1993.

The main housing aim of the British government in 1995 is that a decent home should be within the reach of every family.[a] Current policies are:

1   to promote the growth in owner occupation
2   to encourage the private rented sector
3   to improve performance and value for money in the subsidized sector
4   to direct public expenditure to those most in need of support.

It is by no means clear that expenditure on MITR and housing benefits satisfies policy 3, value for money: in fact, there is a direct contradiction between policy 3 and the trend away from housebuilding and towards housing benefits. Housing benefits are confusing, inequitable and erratic in their effects.

## Help with housing

Housing Benefit is available for tenants, assessed and paid for by local councils. It is available to any tenant with less than £16 000 capital who is on Income Support, whether in or out of work. Income Support (IS) is a benefit for people who are not in remunerative work and whose income is below a minimum level set by parliament.

Income Support for mortgage interest payments is available for the poorest home owners, but only if they do not work. It is paid by the Benefit Agency on behalf of the Department of Social Security. Low-paid workers do not qualify for this benefit. This state of affairs presents some people with the choice of losing their job or losing their home. It was paid to 411 000 people in 1991. People aged over 60 years accounted for 21% of this number, single-parent families 22% and un-employed people 38%. In 1993 £1 billion was paid out in IS for mortgage interest.

Mortgage interest tax relief is administered by the Inland Revenue but is never-theless a subsidy paid to owner-occupiers. As a subsidy, it is extremely poorly tar-geted: £795 million (15% of the total) has been handed out to people earning over £35 000 per year. Over the past 14 years, MITR has cost the taxpayer some £59 billion – enough to build over one million new houses. It is designed to increase owner-occupation, which is not necessarily a bad thing in itself, but in its effects it has been a qualified success. In 1992, 68 540 homes were repossessed, 352 050 households were more than six months in arrears and therefore at risk of repos-session, and one million were in a position of negative equity, in that their mort-gage was more than the value of their house.

[a] The official details in this chapter arise from personal correspondence with the Department of the Environment, for which I am grateful.

## Official homeless management

The Department of the Environment (DoE) reports that use of bed and breakfast accommodation is falling (by 24% in 1993–94) and also that there has been an overall fall of 13% in the number of people in temporary accommodation in the same period, although housing pressure groups believe that this fall at least in part reflects changes in official definitions.

The DoE has written: 'Ministers are not convinced that a significant expansion in public investment in housebuilding...is merited at a time when the Government's priority is to keep public expenditure under control.' (Personal communication.)

The mathematics of the situation indicates that in fact investment in housebuilding is ten times better value for money and that temporary accommodation is a waste of public expenditure. If governments truly wish to realize their main aim, and especially policy 3 on page 90, a major programme of rehabilitation of unfit vacant properties, together with a housebuilding programme, will not only house the homeless and reduce public expenditure in the long run, but also significantly reduce unemployment, poverty and demoralization.

# COST OF TEMPORARY ACCOMMODATION VERSUS COST OF NEW HOUSING

## The cost of temporary accommodation

According to Chartered Institute of Public Finance and Accountability (CIPFA) figures for 1992–93, based on an 83% response to a survey of local authorities, the breakdown of the cost of temporary accommodation is as shown in Table 5.2.

Since this figure represents only 83% of local authorities, it should be increased pro rata to the cost for 100% of local authorities:

$$\frac{419\ 043}{83} \times 100 = £504\ 871.08 \text{ million}$$

This gives a round figure of £504 871 000 for all temporary accommodation in 1992–93. This is a broad estimate, as it depends on an unweighted calculation; the 17% of non-responders might have had a bigger or smaller population than the average.

To put one household in bed and breakfast costs between £12 120 and £13 150 per year, and to put it in private accommodation costs £11 000 per year. Let us take £10 000 as a convenient and conservative figure for keeping one family in temporary accommodation for one year.

**Table 5.2** Cost of temporary accommodation, 1992–93

| Total gross expenditure | (£ million) |
| --- | --- |
| Hostels | 46 033 |
| Bed and breakfast | 118 872 |
| Leasehold dwellings | 167 217 |
| Other | 26 288 |
| Administration and welfare | 60 633 |
| Total | 419 043 |

Source: CIPFA.

Now, if each household costs £10 000 per year, 50 000 households can be provided with a roof for one year by the expenditure of half a billion pounds; in other words, that sum of money purchases 50 000 household-roof-years (HRYs) of temporary accommodation.

# The cost of building social housing

Shelter, the UK national campaigning organization for homeless people, has put out two reports on housebuilding.[2,3] It estimates that, over and above the present programme, 48 000 homes will have to be built each year to satisfy Britain's housing needs. This extra building will cost £1.3 billion per year, and create employment for 120 000 people (Table 5.3).

To the net gain of £404 000 000 per year (£1656 million–£1300 million) could be added savings to the health service resulting from reduced unemployment and homelessness, and to society as a result of reduced alienation.

The cost of building housing that can be afforded by people on low incomes varies from £20 000 to £70 000 (even £150 000 has been quoted for some parts of the country).[2,3] In the West Country, Solon Housing Association considers that it can build one new unit, or buy and refurbish an old unit, for £50 000. Let us take that figure. Assume that the unit would have a lifetime of 100 years. The cost per year of providing that unit of family accommodation is therefore £500 (that is £50 000/100) in capital costs and, if we include £500 per year house maintenance costs, a total of £1000 per HRY. The HRY cost falls with higher quality building that will last longer.

Comparing this with £10 000 per year for putting a family in temporary accommodation, it is ten times more efficient, in strictly financial terms, to build houses for the homeless than to put them up in temporary accommodation. When the health costs of temporary accommodation are included, it becomes even more efficient.

Put another way, to build a house for £50 000 for a homeless family will pay itself back in five years. Over the 100-year lifetime of a house, each unit will pay back 95 × £10 000 = £950 000 in real terms.

**Table 5.3** Balance sheet of the housebuilding equation

| Item | Expenditure (£m) | Income (£m) |
| --- | --- | --- |
| 48 000 units | 1300 | Rent 48 |
| Savings (temporary accommodation costs forgone) | | |
| (48 000 × 12 000) | | 576 |
| Savings in Unemployment Benefit | | |
| (120 000 × 9000) | | 1080 |
| Total | 1300 | 1704 |

# Using empty houses and vacant land

Furthermore, it is not always necessary to spend £50 000 in order to produce a house. A total of 145 000 houses in the UK stand empty, condemned as unfit for human habitation. These houses can be brought back into use at an average cost of only £8400 per unit (see p. 66). If we assume that each refurbished unit has a lifetime of 50 years, the HRY cost is £668, which is:

- only 67% the cost of new building
- 15 times cheaper than temporary accommodation.

Of course, the distribution of unfit houses is not identical to the distribution of homeless households. But if one in three could be brought into use for a local homeless household in this way, some 48 000 homes at £8400 each could be provided for a mere £406 000.

In his book *Homelessness: What Can be Done?*[4] Ron Bailey, the UK Green Party campaign manager, sets out a detailed plan of attack on Britain's housing crisis including a ready-made bill to go before parliament. He makes the case for empty property use orders (EPUOs), which enable local authorities and self-help groups to bring empty properties into use. Ways and means of enabling vacant land to be brought into use are set out, as well as plans for self-build units that could produce a two-bedroom bungalow for £10 000 and a four-bedroom bungalow for £13 700. Finally, he makes a detailed case against the so-called Criminal Justice Act, which has made squatting a criminal action. These low-cost, self-help approaches tip the financial and moral balances even further in favour of providing housing, rather than temporary accommodation, for the homeless.

# The Treasury calculation

Faced with the arguments on the comparative cost-effectiveness of housebuilding as opposed to the provision of temporary accommodation, the government's response is (DoE personal correspondence):

The accepted method of calculating comparative public sector costs is to compare over 30 years rather than one hundred, and to weight costs and benefits so that those which fall in earlier years are relatively more important than those which fall in later years.

Working within a 30-year accounting convention, a £50 000-house costs £1667 per year to buy in capital terms, which is still six times cheaper than temporary accommodation.

The government weighting of earlier years means that in effect the capital must be repaid in eight years. This leads to a HRY cost of £6250, which is still 1.26 times more efficient than temporary accommodation in HRY terms.

Housebuilding only becomes more expensive when the Treasury requires that the full capital cost is shown in the public sector borrowing requirement (PSBR) in the year in which a public sector house is built. For instance, if 48 000 houses were to be built in one year at £50 000, this would be shown as a £2.4 billion increase in the PSBR. This is unconventional accountancy practice. Normal practice in the private sector and throughout the EU would be to register the cost of these houses in that year as the amount of mortgage paid off. For example, if we assume that £50 000 is borrowed over 25 years at 9.5% interest, the annual repayment would be £5300. For the whole 48 000-house programme, the damage to the PSBR is now only £0.25 billion. The Treasury's accounting method inflates the apparent cost of housing by a factor of ten. This, then, is the key to the housing crisis: reality has been overtaken by flaky accountancy. Thousands of families are suffering and being broken up, illness is being generated, building workers are on the dole, construction companies are in recession and investors are being cheated of dividends because of strange accountancy conventions within the Treasury.

There is a solution. It is not likely that more than three chief officials are committed to this accountancy practice. Clearly, their seniority would make it impossible for any chancellor to influence their thinking to any degree. If they could be offered early retirement for, say, one million pounds each, the housing programme could commence within a month. This may be seen as a high-risk strategy, since other officials may develop strange ideas in the hope of benefiting from similar payoffs, but desperate situations require desperate remedies.

# A matter of interest

It may be objected that the costings for housebuilding used above deal with capital alone, and not with the interest. There are three reasons for leaving interest out of the equation:

1   A total of £5.5 billion is lying in the capital receipts funds of local authorities from the sale of council houses, and can be disbursed directly without the need for loans, except between authorities that have more money and those that have more need.

2 If it is necessary to obtain new capital over and above the capital receipt fund, it is not necessary to rely on the banks to create this money. Since this is such a cost-effective investment in financial and socioeconomic terms, the government can use its powers to create the money itself, on zero interest terms. The banks would be creating the new money against the surety of their financial holdings: therefore the government can create the new money against the government's greater financial holdings, and also against the capital resources inherent in the labour, bricks, mortar and wood held by the nation which will be transmuted into a long-lasting capital asset.

3 If option 2 is rejected as too threatening towards the private financial institutions' conventional monopoly on the creation of new money, conventional borrowing would still be more cost-effective than the indefinite use of temporary accommodation for more and more people over the coming century. In the example quoted above, the £5300 mortgage repayment is still cheaper than temporary accommodation.

## Other measures

As well as a national programme of house refurbishment and rebuilding, a spate of reforms are needed to remedy the many problems that we now face. The lack of benefits for young single people prevents them from paying rent: this must be remedied; the problem of the impenetrable labyrinth of helping agencies must be overcome. Deposits must be readily available to allow the homeless to obtain rented lodgings: move-on housing must be provided to cover the gap between hostel and rented accommodation.

## Greening the dismal science

The housing crisis, like the unemployment crisis, is unnecessary; the two problems may to some degree cancel each other out. The fault is not so much in reality (although the continued growth of our population is a real problem that contributes to housing need) as in the conventions we use to view the world. It does not have to be like this.

The problem highlighted in this chapter – that practitioners of the dismal science of economics cannot see the wood of problems in housing reality for the trees of economic theory and conventions – is but one example of the failure of conventional economics to make contact with reality. There is a growing consciousness that economics needs to work from a new framework that is more accurately tied in with the real world. In the UK, the New Economics Foundation is at the forefront of this movement. One of the key issues is the measurement of wealth. New economists argue that the index of wealth of a country must reflect not just its financial assets, but also its natural assets, including such items as environmental degradation, loss of natural capital and social conditions.[5] Figure 5.1 shows the

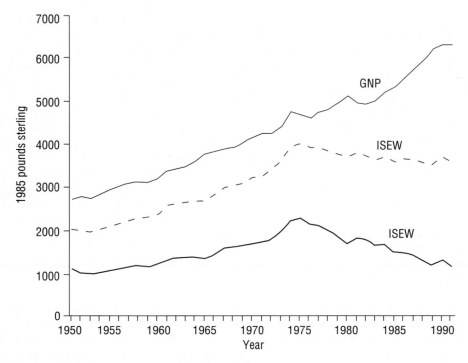

**Figure 5.1** UK ISEW per capita 1950–90. *Dotted line*: excludes contribution of resource depletion and long-term environmental damage. Reproduced with permission from Jackson and Marks.[5] Source: New Economics Foundation.

result for the UK: while the GNP shows a steady rise, the index of sustainable economic welfare (ISEW) shows stagnation.

The key to the change is reckoning with the value of natural assets, instead of classing them as mere 'externalities' to the market. This minor conceptual change carries major implications for our real lives.

For housebuilding, we have the necessary assets:

- resources of human energy and skill (liberated via the wage subsidy)
- bricks (taken from clay and energy capital resources)
- wood, (mainly imported, but increasingly to be harvested in the UK, as the post-war plantings mature)
- capital receipts from council housing scales.

Any necessary new money can be loaned by government at zero interest (or even, if necessary, borrowed conventionally from money created by the banks).

The result of this housebuilding activity is, in the first place, an increased stock of homes. In creating this, our generation would be fulfilling the aim of sustainable development in handing on to future generations a capital resource that is not depleted but enhanced. This is worthwhile in itself, since, despite the lip service paid to sustainable development, we are passing on precious little else in terms of wealth added by this greed-ridden and self-obsessed generation, and a great deal in terms of depleted and contaminated resources.

Over and above this handing on of wealth, we also benefit in real time by incurring:

- less poverty
- less unemployment and more tax revenue
- less illness and therefore increased NHS efficiency, which will contribute to increased economic efficiency with less time lost through illness awaiting treatment
- less crime
- less general demoralization nationwide as the perception grows that something can be done to improve conditions.

The conclusion is therefore that the question is not whether we can afford to build houses, but why we ever thought we could afford not to do so.

## REFERENCES

1    Newton J (1994) *All in One Place (The British Housing Story 1973–1993)*. CHAS (The Catholic Housing Aid Society), London.

2    Foster S (1993) *Missing the Target*. Shelter, London.

3    Shelter (1993) *Supply 100 000 homes, Create jobs*. Shelter Briefing. Shelter, London.

4    Bailey R (1994) *Homelessness: What Can be Done? An Immediate Programme of Self-Help and Mutual Aid*. Jon Carpenter, Oxford.

5    Jackson T and Marks N (1994) *Measuring Sustainable Economic Welfare – A Pilot Index: 1950–1990*. Stockholm Environment Institute, Stockholm.

# 6

# Poverty and
# deprivation

*It's the same the whole world over,*
*It's the poor wot gets the blame*
*It's the rich wot gets the pleasure*
*Ain't it all a bloomin' shame?*

Traditional London song

## INTRODUCTION

Poverty is inextricably interwoven with social class, unemployment, disrupted social conditions and poor housing. It is also admixed with environmental pollution – poor neighbourhoods tend to find themselves, for historic reasons, in the shadow of industrial complexes. Moreover, since these neighbourhoods lack the political clout and articulacy of middle class NIMBY (not in my backyard) groups, they tend to be on the receiving end of waste dumps and other processes not tolerated by other more advantaged communities.

The growing divergence between the monetary incomes of the rich and the poor within nations and between nations is so widespread that it is reasonable to suppose that there is an inherent tendency within the prevailing economic system to bring this about. Clearly, any effort to lessen the impact of poverty, no matter how well intentioned and well executed, is doomed to failure if this tendency is not identified and rectified.

Oscar Lewis, an American anthropologist writing in the 1960s, argued that poverty creates its own self-perpetuating culture characterized by fragile sexual relations, weak family relations, psychological stress and apathy.[1] This 'cycle of deprivation' implies a continuing and increasing disease in society which can only worsen as economic problems brought about by environmental degradation begin to bite. Radical steps must be taken to redistribute income equitably.

## POVERTY AND HAPPINESS

A survey of Illinois residents in 1965 asked people to classify themselves as 'very happy', 'pretty happy' or 'not too happy'. The results are shown in Figure 6.1 a and b, which plot the percentage of responses in each category against level of income. Figure 6.1a shows that most people class themselves as 'pretty happy', with fewer at the extremes of poverty and wealth. Few of the poor, and more of the rich, rated themselves as 'very happy'. More of the poor classed themselves as 'not too happy'.[2]

In Figure 6.1b the assessments have been lumped together by giving 'very happy' a score of two, 'pretty happy' a score of one and 'not too happy' a score of

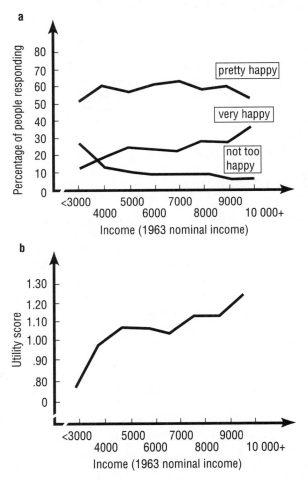

**Figure 6.1** Income and happiness. **a** Survey results. **b** Utility score. The utility scores are the averages for each income category if 'very happy' is assigned a value of +2, 'pretty happy' a value of +1 and 'not too happy' a value of 0. Source:[2].

zero. This suggests that people's self-rating of happiness rises with wealth, with a marked fall-off into misery for those on lowest incomes.

## DEFINITIONS OF POVERTY

Deprivation itself has many facets beyond income poverty: Chambers[3] points to weakness, social isolation, inferiority, powerlessness, humiliation and vulnerability as additional factors that, although difficult to measure, are very powerful agents in people's experience. Johda found that farmers and villagers in Rajasthan, India, when asked to give their own criteria for economic status tended to give lower priority to monetary wealth than to real conditions such as disablement, lack of land, livestock and farm equipment, difficulty in getting a decent burial and so on.[4] He found 36 households were worse off in monetary income, but better off by their own criteria.

This situation is more likely to apply in agricultural societies, in which wealth comes from land, than in our urban societies where money is all-important, but it does serve to remind us that monetary wealth is a only a limited indicator of real wealth, and it confirms the Index of Sustainable Economic Welfare (ISEW) approach outlined in chapter 5. The term 'poverty' is usually taken to mean low financial income, whereas 'deprivation' covers the wider aspects.

Given the need to apply a measuring rod to the complex phenomenon of deprivation, we can go about it in two ways: as relative poverty or as absolute poverty.

## Relative poverty

Relative poverty in a population is usually defined as income (or, more precisely, the income adjusted for household size and after taking account of housing costs) that is below 50% of the average income level. In 1991 the average income was £61.33 per week for a single person and £160.56 for a couple with two children aged six and eight years.

The British government does not officially recognize this definition, arguing that, as average income goes up, so does the number of people below the poverty line, so that the definition of poverty is invalidated. This ignores the fact that the motive behind an increase in the average income is to keep pace with inflation. If the average keeps in-step with inflation, 50% of the average is by definition falling behind inflation, thus increasing the numbers in poverty.

Ministers argue further that if Income Support is used as a benchmark, then each time it is increased the number of those who are defined as in poverty also increases. This argument is somewhat academic since, in real terms, Income Support has not increased, but decreased (see p. 103). The Income Support argument of the government to the relative poverty index may be avoided by taking the level of half of the national average wage in 1979 as the standard. On this count, the numbers in poverty still increased, and the number living in poverty and whose family is unemployed doubled from 800 000 to 1 600 000.

The validity of relative poverty as an index is supported by evidence from the examination of health rates in relation to relative poverty. Wilkinson[5] has followed up accepted cross-sectional evidence which has shown that there is a significant tendency for mortality rates to be lower in countries with a more equitable distribution of income. He confirmed these findings by showing that, as time passed, the average change in percentage share of the total income of a country was positively related to changes in life expectancy. In other words, countries that were, over the years, distributing their wealth more equally tended to have better levels of health. In particular, Japan, with most egalitarian tendencies in distribution of wealth (let us call this a 'convergent economy') obtained the best decrease in mortality rate, whereas the UK, with the greatest changes towards inequality (which we may call a 'divergent economy'), fared worst of all. The other four comparable countries were strung inbetween these two extremes, confirming that the relationship was proportional.

Wilkinson[6] has also shown a relationship between relative poverty and life expectancy, infant mortality, suicide in men aged 15–24, depression, crime rates and decline in reading standards.

The conclusion is that relative poverty is a relevant and valid index. The number of individuals who earn half of the average income has risen:

| | | |
|------|-------------|------------------------------|
| 1979 | 5 million   | 9% of the UK population      |
| 1991 | 13.5 million| 24% of the UK population.    |

The fact that nearly one-quarter of our citizens live in relative poverty is not one that we can be proud of as a nation.

Does the economic divergence cause the ill-health or are both factors perhaps related to a third common factor? While 'proof', as ever, is not available, our understanding of several factors set out below is enough to give a reasonable expectation that if the British economy changed towards a convergent mode, the health of the poorer part of the nation would improve.

## Absolute poverty

Robert MacNamara, a former President of the World Bank, defined absolute poverty as:

> A condition of life so limited by malnutrition, illiteracy, disease, squalid surroundings, high infant mortality and low life expectancy as to be beneath any reasonable definition of human decency.

Clearly, few people in the UK qualify for this definition of poverty, although the qualitative statement 'reasonable definition of human decency' leaves the door open for debate as to where the line might be drawn. Nevertheless, absolute poverty is a useful concept even in the UK, if it is related to the means to obtain the basic necessities of life.

Absolute poverty can be measured by costing the necessities of life. The Family Budget Unit (FBU) uses a 'budget standards' method, costing a range of goods and services that are deemed to be necessary for bringing about living standards that are acceptable as a modern minimum. The method considers detailed factors such as the fact that the 18–25 year age group has increased nutritional needs compared with other age groups. (Contrast this with the falling income support levels which have been extended to this age group, as detailed below.)

On this basis, at 1994 prices, a couple with two children would need £140 per week. Compare this with the actual benefit levels for 1994, set at £71.70: approximately half of that which the Family Budget Unit calculates to be necessary. Similarly the FBU level for a child stands at £25 per week: the actual benefit received is £15.65.

Unemployment creates poverty. Between 1979 and 1991 the proportion of the poorest tenth of the UK population which was unemployed grew from 16% to 28%. In 1991 72% of families in which the head of the household was unemployed had an income that was half or below half of the average income.

Social Security benefits have been falling relative to average earnings. Between 1979 and 1993 the benefit for a single person fell from 23% of the net income of an average home owner to only 17.4%: for a married couple, it fell from 36% to 27%. Income Support, which is a benefit paid to people whose income is below a minimum level set by parliament, has fallen in real terms for a young (18–24) single person from £42.70 to £34.80 over this period – a cut of more than one-fifth.

The common definition of poverty is the state that a person is in when receiving Income Support. Townsend[7] found that financial difficulties sufficient to cause social problems continue until people reach at least 40% more than the Income Support level. By convention, the level between IS and IS +40% is referred to as low income.

# Indicators of deprivation

Social class (Table 6.1), as defined in the Registrar General's classification of occupations, is usually used as a rough indicator of which groups are likely to be deprived and which are not. The relationship between social class and poverty is gradually becoming blurred as society changes. Home ownership, second incomes, single parenthood and unemployment are cutting across the traditional relationship between husband's occupation and family's income, so that social scientists are now trying to develop alternative socioeconomic indicators.

Osborne and Morris included in their assessment of social class educational achievement of parents, quality of housing, degree of overcrowding, income and availability of the use of a car.[8] Only social and family relationships are left out of the assessment. This method will certainly bring deprivation into much clearer focus, but at the expense of making assessments far more difficult to make.

**Table 6.1**  Social class

| | |
|---|---|
| I | Professional, e.g. surveyor |
| II | Intermediate, e.g. musician, farmer |
| IIIN | Skilled non-manual, e.g. clerical |
| IIIM | Skilled manual, e.g. bricklayer, driver |
| IV | Partly skilled, e.g. barperson, gardener |
| V | Unskilled, e.g. labourer |

Instead of using the characteristics of the individual as the starting point of mea-surement, several methods have been developed that use instead the character-istics of the area that the individual comes from. The results of these methods do not yet agree with each other, but a standard will no doubt emerge eventually, since knowledge of the attributes of an area are of practical importance to plan-ning of health, social services and economic development.

The area method appears to work even at a level as broad as the regions of the UK. Regional unemployment figures give useful data about the probability of car crime and single parenthood (Figures 2.2 and 6.2).

Recently, it has been suggested that the proportion of prescriptions in an area which is exempt from prescription charges can act as a simple indicator of depri-

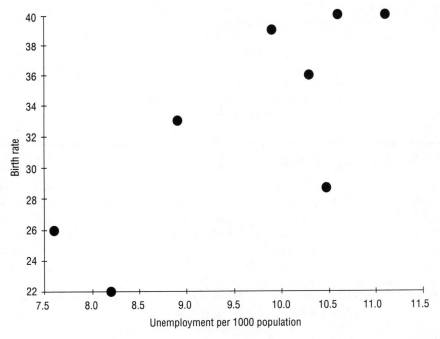

**Figure 6.2**   Unemployment versus <20 year birth rate, by UK region. Source: Regional Trends.

vation. It has the great advantage of being up-to-date, as statistics on prescription charges are collected quarterly, rather than every decade for the census.

# THE EFFECTS OF POVERTY ON HEALTH

## Mortality and morbidity

Socioeconomic status is a powerful predictor of mortality.[9] A recent paper in the *BMJ*[10] concludes that current targets for reducing coronary heart disease mortality may be achievable if the mortality in poor areas can be reduced to the rates in affluent areas. A person who lives in an inner city area is likely to die eight years before a similar person in other areas.

Infant mortality is clearly related to poverty. Post-neonatal mortality (that is any death that occurs between 28 weeks and 12 months) is 2.7 times higher for children born into social class V than those born into social class I.

Mortality from all causes in children aged one year or under is 2.2 times higher in poorer families. Children in unskilled manual homes are 1.5 times more likely to die in the first year of life.

A study for Sheffield Health Authority has shown that people who live in the inner city have more than twice the risk of dying prematurely from coronary heart disease compared to the average person.[11] The health gap between rich and poor had widened over a period of eight years according to the study.

## Accidents

The Health of the Nation strategy has established the prevention of accidents as a key area or national priority. This is because, as death rates from infections fall due to better medical care, accidents have now emerged as the leading cause of death in younger age groups. If we look at childhood accidents, children living in poverty are clearly the group most at risk. Mortality from injuries in under-15-year-olds is 3.8 times higher in poorer families than in better-off families. The chance of children from unskilled manual homes dying in a road traffic accident is four times higher and their chance of dying in a fire is six times higher.

In any programme of improvement, it is important to start at the point where the greatest improvement is to be made. Surprisingly, the *Department of Health Key Area Handbook*[12] on accidents, in its detailed advice on accident prevention, makes no reference to targeting lower income families. This aspect appears only as an oblique reference to research on the effect socioeconomic factors have on the prevention of accidents. This is a perplexing omission.

Since poverty-stricken families are least able to take on board well-meant accident prevention advice, partly because of lower levels of education and partly because of their pervading sense of powerlessness, it is useless to target them with an avalanche of literature, or even with intensified visits from health visitors. For any programme to have an impact on accidents, it will be necessary at the same time to take action to relieve the conditions of deprivation itself.

# Child abuse

Child abuse is classified into these groups:

- physical injury
- sexual
- neglect
- emotional
- failure to thrive
- neglect and physical
- physical and sexual
- grave concern.

Any child who is known to the authorities as being at risk of abuse is placed on a register. Dr Susan Creighton of the NSPCC[13] comments that:

> the parents of the registered children were much less likely to be in paid employment than parents nationally ... The parents of non-organic failure to thrive, N+P (neglect and physical abuse) and neglect cases were the least likely to be in paid employment. The parents most likely to be in employment were those of physically injured and sexually abused children.

In looking at the social class of parents of children on the at-risk register, it was found that there were so few parents in professional and intermediate occupations that it was necessary to group them with group IIIN into a general non-manual category, which formed 4–5% of the total.[13] It is, of course, possible that people in these groups are more skilled at hiding their abuse, less likely to be suspected or more able to avoid investigation and prosecution. This category showed the greatest likelihood of physically or sexually abusing the children in their care and the least likelihood of having children who were suffering failure to thrive or neglect.

Since this is a cross-sectional survey, it is not possible to infer much about the causation of abuse from these facts, beyond noting that the increased poverty associated with being unemployed is consistent with failure to thrive. The finding that physical and sexual abuse is associated with employed 'parents' in the higher grades of occupation is unexpected. It is possible to speculate that the frustrations generated by poor patterns of work are being taken out on the children.

Despite the explosion of press stories about sexual abuse in childhood, it does not seem that levels in society now are any different from those found in the 1940s. Paediatricians from Ottowa studied the Kinsey Report of 1953 and made comparisons with recent studies.[14] They found that the rate of sexual abuse (sadly 10–12% of girls younger than 14 years) was the same in all studies.

## Stomach ulcers

It has long been known that stomach ulcers and stomach cancers are associated with poverty. Areas with high rates of stomach cancer in north-west Wales are associated with high rates of overcrowding in the past.[15]

Recent work has led to the conclusion that stomach ulcers, hyperacidity and stomach cancers are caused by an organism called *Helicobacter pylori*. Increased transmission of this organism as a result of overcrowding would account for the Wales findings.

## Deprivation and infectious disease

### Tuberculosis

Tuberculosis (TB) has always been associated with poverty, and the incidence of the disease had been falling steadily until recently. The decline began in the late nineteenth century, before the advent of chemotherapy (effective medication), and this decline is generally accepted to have been due to improvements in housing and diet. The decline has now stopped, and the incidence is actually increasing in the UK[16] and the USA. This increase is influenced in the USA by the spread of AIDS, but the increase in the UK is not caused in this way, since it is much greater than could be accounted for by HIV. Only about 2% of TB patients (aged 16–54) in the UK are HIV positive. By comparison, two-thirds of TB patients in Zambia have AIDS.

It is possible that deprivation may contribute to the spread of TB: overcrowded accommodation increases transmission rates, and protein undernutrition causes alteration in T-cell reaction. T-cells are members of the immune system which fight tubercle bacilli. Spence *et al*.[17] in 1993 conducted a study in Liverpool, looking back over past case notes. They found that TB rates corresponded closely with all measures of deprivation, and that the rates were independent of ethnic groups. They pointed to the possibility that, as HIV infection becomes more common, TB in that group will also increase in the UK as it has in the USA.

In Caucasian groups, the pattern at the moment is that the cases which are being found are caused by a reactivation of old TB. The rates for this reactivation have been found to be higher in a poor area of Leeds.[18] Poor housing was a feature of an outbreak of tuberculosis in Leeds in which 18 children and three adults were infected.[19]

Two reports in the *BMJ* support the impression that increasing rates of poverty are contributing to the increase in TB. One[20] compared TB notification levels and unemployment, overcrowding, social class and immigrants in 32 London boroughs. It was found that notifications were positively associated with overcrowding and the proportion of immigrants in an area. There was a weak positive association with the rate of change in notifications and the rate of increase in unemployment, which explained 25% of the TB rate. A second report[21] that examined the rate of TB in 403 districts in the UK found that the rate of increase was 35% in the poorest tenth of the population, 13% in the next two-tenths and nil in the richest 70%. In Hackney, it was found that TB among recent immigrants could explain only half of the observed increase.

The conclusion is that the increase in relative and absolute poverty in recent years is responsible for half of the increase in TB. Moreover, the presence of an undernourished underclass in the UK (vulnerable to TB infection) offers an opening to the larger threat which is presented by the emergence of drug-resistant strains of TB bacillus in less developed countries. Inadequate combinations of drugs which are sometimes prescribed in those lands allow the bacillus to survive and to learn how to destroy the drugs. Concentrations of drug-resistant strains have reached Barcelona already.

## Recommendations

1  the UK should respond to the WHO appeal for money to fight TB, should subscribe to the International Union against Tuberculosis and Lung Disease and should increase its £11 million budget for TB research

2  measures to break the poverty trap and improve the standard for housing should be set in place in order to stop the increase in TB and protect our population against resistant strains.

## Tuberculosis treatment

The cost of the drugs required to treat one patient with a standard course of isoniazid and rifampicin for six months, together with pirazinide for two months initially, comes to £516.

Assuming that each patient requires six outpatients appointments over a year of successfully completed treatment at £40 per appointment, add £240.

Add three chest radiographs at £10 each = £30.

The total cost of treating one patient is therefore £786.

If the total number of 'extra' cases per year is 1000 (that is cases over and above those that would have occurred had the previous rate of decline continued), then the total cost of treating 'extra' cases = £786 000.

## Other infectious diseases

Respiratory illness is increased in deprived conditions. A child of five years old in a poor family is more likely to have had pneumonia than the average, and twice as likely to die of respiratory illness.[22]

Other infections are also associated with deprivation. Typhoid incidence is higher in deprived areas, as is *Shigella sonnei* dysentery. The health cost of this form of dysentery has been estimated to be £40 311 for 144 confirmed cases of dysentery.[23] Extrapolating to the 9830 cases that occurred in England and Wales in 1993 gives a total cost of £2 751 786. The incidence of *Shigella sonnei* dysentery has risen fourfold in two years.

The manifestations of *Streptococcus* infections are suspected to interact with stress. In one study, a group of people who were known to carry *Streptococcus* were followed. Those who were stressed became ill; those who were not stressed did not.[24] However, this work has not yet been replicated.

# WHY DOES POVERTY AFFECT HEALTH?

Three main agents are suggested to be the cause of ill-health in deprived populations: malnutrition, fuel poverty and psychosocial factors.

## Poor diet

We have seen that the Family Budget Unit has shown that Income Support is inadequate to buy good food. Confirmatory evidence that people in social class V are malnourished comes from the fact that both children and adults from this class are smaller in stature, and it is known that undernutrition can bring this about. Undernutrition in childhood can also cause apathy and withdrawal.[25]

Paradoxically, more people in social classes IV and V are overweight. This is because the cheapest way of avoiding hunger is to eat low-quality, high-calorie fatty foods. Poor people also eat more refined carbohydrates (sugar), but fewer vitamins and minerals.[26] The manual classes also suffer more from ischaemic heart disease and caries. Ischaemic heart disease is believed to be caused by fat, and caries is known to be caused by sugar.

Poor diet, with marginal deficiencies of proteins, vitamins and minerals, impairs the ability of the immune system. Protein deficiency is known to enable the reactivation of old tuberculosis. Vitamin and mineral deficiencies may combine with overcrowding and other environmental conditions to cause susceptibility to viral and bacterial infections, as well as general lethargy and relative incompetence of the immune system.

Elderly people, especially the poor elderly, are known to suffer dietary deficiency. Since they do not move about as much as younger people, their appetites are less. Eating less of poor-quality food results in deficiency in minerals and vitamins. A wise saying current among general practitioners is 'Next to loneliness, the chief enemy of the elderly is vitamin deficiency'.

# Fuel poverty

In chapter 4 the effects of low temperature on health are set out. Eight million households live in fuel poverty. Members of each of these households will develop illness related to damp and cold, and if we assume that the cost to the NHS of treating these illnesses is £100 per person per year – an extremely conservative assumption – the total annual cost to the NHS is £800 million.

## Mortality and ambient temperature

Peter Woodhouse[27] has shown that when elderly people are exposed to cold their blood pressure rises. This will tend to cause strokes, and may explain some of the extra mortality that occurs after cold spells. Alternatively, if their GP happens to identify the raised blood pressure, they may be started on antihypertensive medication. This carries a cost implication to the NHS, and for a few may lead to side-effect problems.

# Psychosocial effects

It has not proved possible to lay the cause of the observed poor health seen in those who are deprived at the door of any known cause such as smoking or cholesterol. In the absence of this, the agreed hypothetical explanation is that the cause is 'psychosocial', a vague term which implies that the societal position affects the psyche, which in turn affects the physical health of the individual. Models for these effects are known from primate studies and psychoneuroimmunology. An anecdote may help to cover our deficiency in the precise details of psychosocial processes. A consultant physician coming up to retirement age noted with surprise that his choice of year to leave was the first major life choice he had made since he had decided to become a doctor. He had made thousands of important professional choices regarding his patients, naturally, but his own life had run on smooth rails. Compare this with a mother on Income Support who weekly has to decide whether to pay the gas bill or the rent bill, choices which are immediate and personal, affecting the well-being of her family, and choices which are going to hurt whichever path she selects. It is perhaps in this weekly agonizing over matters of security which wears the deprived so heavily.

# SPECIAL ASPECTS OF POVERTY

# Social deprivation

To be poor is to be locked out of twentieth century society. Everywhere surrounded by advertisements using sophisticated techniques to persuade them to buy this, have that, desire the other, the result is a feeling of shame and inadequacy. Middle-class parents who are taken aback at the drive of their children to possess the best – witness the fashion for expensive trainers in the late 1980s – can only imagine the pain and sense of exclusion of parents who cannot satisfy the 'needs' induced by advertising.

## Population increase

Unemployment is associated with men with larger families, and the number of large families affected by unemployment is rising faster than the number of smaller families (Table 6.2).

Does unemployment cause people to have more children? Certainly there is ample time during the unemployed day for parents to make love. One possibility is that a small baby adds joy to an otherwise empty life. For a person in a dependent position at the bottom of the social pecking order, there is an incentive to have a small, perfect, lovable dependent person to look after. The fact that the small, gurgling baby is also a cause of sleep deprivation and rapidly turns into an unruly independent source of trouble and worry as well as love is not something that gets consideration well in advance of the event.

Figure 6.2 shows the relationship between unemployment by region and pregnancies among women below the age of 20. A positive relationship is suggested. The graph of unemployment rates with children placed in care, again on a regional basis (Figure 6.3), also suggests a positive association. Certainly the hypothesis that unemployment and poverty cause more teenage pregnancies and placements of children into care needs testing.

Of the industrialized western nations, the teenage conception rate in the UK is among the highest, being second only to the USA. Denmark, France, The Netherlands and Switzerland have the lowest rates. Whereas in most other nations teenage conception rates fell considerably between 1980 and 1990, our rates have varied little in that time, and are now showing a rising trend.

Educational attainment and social class are factors known to be determinants of teenage motherhood.[28] The lower the educational attainment, the greater the risk of teenage pregnancy: and the more manual the social class of the father (when recorded), the greater the risk. In fact, for a number of reasons it is difficult to allocate social class accurately to women. The connection can be double-checked using the area method. First, the problem relates to inner cities: rates for women between 13–15 and 15–19 are lowest in mixed urban–rural and highest in inner London and the metropolitan districts. Even using the crudest, regional data,

**Table 6.2** Male unemployment according to number of children

|  | No children (%) | Three or more children (%) |
|---|---|---|
| 1979 | 2 | 6 |
| 1990 | 3 | 10 |

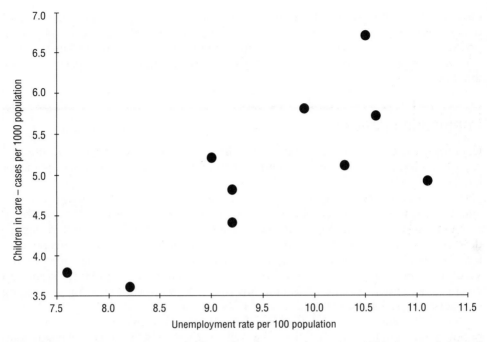

**Figure 6.3** Unemployment versus children placed in care, by region, 1992. Source: Regional Trends.

unemployment at regional level shows a proportional relationship with teenage pregnancies (see Figure 6.2).

It seems reasonable to draw the conclusion that if society wishes to halt population growth (which it must in the name of sustainability) and to reduce the number of teenage pregnancies (which is a Health of the Nation target), more resources must be put into education and into overcoming poverty and unemployment.

## Multiple deprivation and the underclass

Social scientists have been scratching their heads on the question of whether unemployment and poverty are in the process of, or in danger of, giving rise to an underclass. It is a nice philosophical problem, bringing with it difficulties of definition, measurement and what it means in practical terms if they do actually arrive at the conclusion that an underclass exists.

The key feature according to Dahrendorf[29] is that the underclass develops a lifestyle 'which has little in common with the values of a work society around'. Much of the study of the underclass has been carried out in the USA,[30] possibly because the social diseases of racism, drugs and violent crime are further developed in that country. Murray[31] identified male illegitimacy, crime and unemployment as the key features of the underclass.

Writings about the underclass are notably short on measurement and statistics. One statistic that does stand out, however, is the remarkable dip in the numbers of young men that appeared in the 1991 census which followed the abortive introduction of the poll tax. This census 'missed' some 1.2 million people, half of them young adults. Twenty per cent of men in inner London did not respond, and non-response rates were also high in other metropolitan areas.

It is thought that a large number of young men avoided filling in the census forms out of fear that their whereabouts would be traced by local council poll tax collectors.[32] These young men will tend to have no formal statistical identity, or will create false identities for the purposes of collecting benefit. They are alienated from the machinery of state. They will be less likely to have a true formal identity in official dealings and more likely to assume false identities. They are prime candidates for underclass status.

The confusion of social scientists about the nature, existence and meaning of underclass is understandable, given the nature of the subject. Heisenger postulated that the presence of the physicist or, more accurately, the act of looking, would affect the behaviour of subatomic particles. How much more so the effect of the social scientist on an underclass. It is no easy task to administer social attitudes questionnaires to people who regard anyone asking questions as a cop until proved otherwise. Hostility to any representative of 'straight' society, and absolute suspicion of anything to do with science or measurement, will not help the labours of would-be students of the underclass. The very notion of the study is treated with scorn by candidates for underclass status (personal communication). Their reaction could be summarized as:

> Of course there is an underclass. We are not part of that violence out there – the tarmac, the buildings, the motor car, the arms sales, the corruption, the consumerism.

They point to the Criminal Justice Act, which they perceive as a direct assault on their right to demonstrate peacefully and to associate and travel freely, and to regulations in the Job Seekers' Allowance which mean that if they do not assume a conventional appearance they will lose their benefit. The only meaningful change which they seek is revolution, an ill-defined cataclysm which exists only as an undeveloped idea. Any reform of the present system is seen only as a rearranging of the deckchairs on the *Titanic*.

A survey by the Policy Studies Institute of 2400 16 to 17-year-olds from England's inner cities, many in full-time education,[33] showed a deep distrust of the police and criminal justice system.

Only 8% of blacks and 25% of whites thought that courts gave everyone 'fair and equal treatment'. Forty per cent of the boys had been stopped by police for questioning at least once in the previous year. For blacks the figure was 50%. Eighteen per cent of the boys who had been stopped reported 11 or more such incidents.

The same survey showed that faith in democracy is fading. Sixteen per cent of blacks and 12% of whites saw no point in voting. This point is made over and over again by young people: there is no point in voting. When significant numbers of young people find themselves without faith in the system of justice and without faith in the normal channels of changing the system, the likelihood is that at some point they will vent their discontent in outbursts of violence, as indeed happens from time to time as first one then another inner city minority explodes over some 'last straw' piece of perceived or real provocation.

The characteristic mood of the underclass is hostility to all that is part of the present system. In practical terms, the notion of whether or not there is an under-class is an academic irrelevance; what is of importance to us all is the real, existent sense of hostile alienation. It is this mood which should be taken note of and addressed, and only in such a way that we can understand fully its roots and make societal changes designed to prevent its further development.

The first step on the long road to reintegrating this disaffected generation should be to extend an amnesty to non-payers of the poll tax. Since, in the main, these people have no money, the cost of this measure, especially when set against the administrative costs of hunting them down and the total cost of the poll tax exercise itself (set at £19 billion), would be negligible.

A further measure that must be considered to bring the underclass back into the fold is the decriminalization of cannabis.

This may seem a perverse notion, given the association between crime and drugs referred to in chapter 2 on unemployment, but it is a question of the direction of causation: does cannabis use lead to use of harder drugs and therefore crime, or does the fact that the law makes no distinction between cannabis, heroin and crack cocaine tend to expose the cannabis user to a criminal subculture?

Twenty-five years ago, the argument against cannabis was that is was a new phenomenon that must be stamped out before it took hold. One generation later, this strategy has clearly failed, and professionals in the field, most notably senior police officers, have admitted that they have lost the war against cannabis. Like it or not, we must accept the fact that cannabis is established as a recreational drug in the UK, as it is in many countries of the world. The question therefore is not whether it can be eradicated – it cannot – but which is the best way for society to adjust to the new situation. Clearly, to continue to regard aficionados of this weed as criminals *per se*, and to arrest them, try them and imprison them, is helping neither to win the war against drug use nor society to be at peace with itself. The legal situation creates glaring anomalies: drunkenness is used successfully in court as a defence for those who commit serious acts of violence, whereas cannabis intoxication, which generally leads to a state of benignly passive inertia, is in the eyes of the law a crime in and of itself. The second anomaly is that physicians are not at present (1995) allowed to use cannabis even in research despite the mounting evidence that it is beneficial in treatment of the disabling and painful spasms of multiple sclerosis, although we routinely use the addictive drug heroin in treatment of pain.

The cost of the underclass phenomenon must be measured in terms of the policing of demonstrations and insurance costs to deal with riots and civil disorder. For instance, the Home Office admitted in December 1994 that the protests against the M11 link road in east London, when non-violent direct action by environmental activists and locals held up the demolition of houses and the uprooting of trees for weeks, had cost £2 million in policing costs. The costs of outright rebellion would run to one or two orders of magnitude more than this.

## Effects of poverty on education

The English educational system is marked by its reliance on passing academic examinations as a token of education. The effect of this is that those leaving school without any examination success are marked as failures, which may result in lifelong loss of confidence and self-esteem. Before the introduction of the GCSE, as many as 10% of school leavers were stigmatized in this way.

Learning ability is a result of genetic and environmental factors. Slow cognitive development and poor educational progress in preschool and school-age children are associated with socioeconomic deprivation.[34] Poor diet is likely to play a large part in this deficit. The disadvantage is likely to follow those affected throughout life, and also to be transmitted to the next generation. Over and above the direct effects, people affected in this way are less likely to be able to understand health promotional literature and advice.

## THE COST OF POVERTY TO THE NHS

Precision is impossible in costing poverty because of the problem with exact definitions of the population at risk, but as there is no reasonable doubt that poverty and deprivation do cause increased illness there will certainly be a cost penalty to the NHS, and it is possible to reach an estimate from standardized mortality ratios (SMRs) of populations affected by poverty, and from the SMRs to use standard official tables used in calculating resource allocations within the NHS.

Phillimore[35] gives tables relating income levels to SMR [Table II] which show that the most deprived fifth of the population has a mortality rate 50% higher than the average and that, for the next group up, mortality is 20% higher. These figures are for the north of England, where wealth inequalities are more marked and therefore health inequalities will also be more extreme. If we assume conservatively that the lowest quarter of the population (who fall into the definition of relative poverty) have an SMR of 1.20, it is possible to estimate the increased need for resources since standard NHS tables show that a population with an SMR of 1.20 should receive an allocation 9.5% more than the average: 9.5% × 25% = 2.38% and 2.38% of £40 245 million (1992 estimated NHS budget) = £957 831 000.

Since the numbers in poverty and the severity of poverty have increased since 1979, this burden on the NHS has increased. Phillimore's table shows that the SMR for the most deprived tenth of the population has increased by 158–145 = 13%, and for the most deprived fifth by 150–136 = 14% between 1981 and 1989. Taking a 10% increase to accommodate the more severe conditions produced in the northern region, and referring again to the standard tables, a 10% increase in SMR calls for a 4.9% increase in resourcing. If this is applied to 25% of the population, it follows that the increase in poverty since 1979 may be equivalent to a cut in NHS funding of $4.9 \times 25\% = 1.2\%$.

## CONCLUSION

Just as we cannot afford unemployment and homelessness, so also we cannot afford poverty. Although the divergence between rich and poor within nations and between nations is a common tendency, it is not necessary: some nations are achieving convergence. If we do not do so, the outlook is grim, as our already sleazy social fabric begins to give way under the strain. Trickle-down is, and always was, a fantasy: minimum wage is of no benefit for those who are not in work: the only realistic way forward is through citizen's income and a direct Keynesian attack on the conditions that are threatening us: homelessness and environmental degradation.

## REFERENCES

1   Lewis O (1976) *Five Families: Mexican Case Studies in the Culture of Poverty.* Souvenir Press, London.

2   Byrns R T and Stone G W (1989) *Economics.* Scott Foresman and Co., Glenview, Illinois and London.

3   Chambers R (1994) *Poverty and Livelihoods: whose reality counts?.* Overview paper for the Stockhom Roundtable on Global Change, Stockholm.

4   Johda N S (1988) Poverty Debate in India: a Minority View. *Economic and Political Weekly.* **Special Number**: 2421–8.

5   Wilkinson R G (1992) Income Distribution and Life Expectancy. *BMJ*. **304**; 165–8.

6   Wilkinson R G (1994) *Unfair Shares.* Barnardo's, London.

7   Townsend P (1979) *Poverty in the UK.* Penguin, London.

8   Osborne A F and Morris T C (1979) The rationale for a composite index of social class and its evaluation. *Br J Sociology*: **30(1)**; 39–60.

9   Marmot M G, Shipley M J, Rose G (1984) Inequalities of death – specific explanations of a general pattern? *Lancet*: **i**; 1003–6.

10  Eames M, Ben-Schlomo Y, Marmot M G (1993) Social deprivation and premature mortality: regional comparison across England. *BMJ*: **307**; 1097–102.

11 Snell P (1995) *A Health Profile of Sheffield's Electoral Wards.* Sheffield Health Authority, Sheffield.

12 Department of Health (1995) *Department of Health Key Area Handbook.* Department of Health, London.

13 NSPCC (1992) *Child Abuse Trends in England and Wales 1988–1990.* NSPCC, London.

14 Feldman W, Feldman E, Goodman J T *et al.* (1991) Is childhood sexual abuse really increasing in prevalence? An analysis of the evidence. *Paediatrics:* **88(1)**; 29–33.

15 Barker D J P, Coggon D, Osmond C *et al.* (1990) Poor housing in childhood and high rates of stomach cancer in England and Wales. *Br J Cancer:* **61**; 575–8.

16 OPCS (1991) *Communicable Diseases 1987–1990. Series MB2, No. 14–17.* HMSO, London.

17 Spence D P, Hotchkiss C S D, Davies P D O (1993) Tuberculosis and poverty. *BMJ:* **307**; 1143.

18 Kearney M T, Warklyn P D, Teale C *et al.* (1993) Tuberculosis and poverty. *BMJ:* **307**; 1143.

19 Teale C, Cundall D B, Pearson S B (1991) Outbreak of tuberculosis in a poor urban community. *J Infect:* **23**; 327–9.

20 Mangatani P, Jolley D J, Watson J M *et al.* (1995) Socioeconomic deprivation and notification rates for tuberculosis in London during 1982–91. *BMJ:* **310**; 963–6.

21 Bhatti N, Law M R, Morris J K (1995) Increasing incidence of tuberculosis in England and Wales: a study of the likely causes. *BMJ:* **310**; 967–9.

22 Townsend P and Davidson N (eds) (1982) *The Black Report.* Penguin, London.

23 Creedon J and Murphy G (1993) Economic Impact of Dysentry. *Environ Health:* **June**; 176–9.

24 Meyer R and Haggerty R J (1962) Streptococcal infections in families – factors altering susceptibility. *Pediatrics:* **29**; 539–50.

25 Goldbloom R B (1986) 'Failure to Thrive. In: A Demirjian and M Dubuc (eds) *Human Growth: a Multidisciplinary Review.* Taylor and Francis, London.

26 Cole-Hamilton I and Lang T (1986) *Tightening belts: a report on the impact of poverty on food.* London Food Commission, London.

27 Woodhouse P (1993) Seasonal variation of blood pressure and relation to ambient temperature in elderly population. *J Hypertens:* **11(11)**; 1267–74.

28 Babb P (1993) Teenage Conceptions and Fertility in England and Wales, 1971–91. *OPCS Population Trends 74.* Government Statistical Service, London.

29 Dahrendorf R (1987) The erosion of citizenship and its consequences for us all. *New Statesman.*

30 Wilson W J (1987) *The Truly Disadvantaged: The Inner City, The Underclass, and Public Policy.* University of Chicago Press, Chicago.

**31**  Murray C (1990) *The Emerging British Underclass.* IEA Health and Welfare Unit, London.

**32**  Dorling D and Simpson S (1993) Those missing millions: implications for social statistics of undercount in the 1991 census. *Radical Stat.* **55**; 14–35.

**33**  *Changing Lives 3*, BEBC Distribution, Poole, Dorset.

**34**  Fogelman K (1983) *Growing up in Great Britain.* Macmillan, London.

**35**  Phillimore P, Beattie A, Townsend P (1994) Widening inequality of health in northern England, 1981–91. *BMJ.* **308**; 1125–9.

# 7

# Impact of global environmental issues on health

*Why should I care about posterity? What's posterity ever done for me?*

Marx (Groucho)

## INTRODUCTION

The 'environment' is everything. Not only does it comprise everything outside ourselves, but also our body is a 'milieu internal', a self-regulating environment. Human beings as a species form an important part of the environment for other living things. The issues that form part of 'environmentalism' are as large as the planet itself, and include long-term, worldwide problems such as population growth, nuclear proliferation and militarism, climate change, soil erosion, resource depletion and ozone layer thinning, as well as problems closer to home, such as air pollution, water pollution and waste disposal. All of these have an effect on our health that is detectable now, but for our descendants the impacts will become graver as the decades pass. If we were to include within our present national accounts a figure for the impact of our habits on our descendants' health, the figure would doubtless make the national debt look trivial by comparison. Because the subject is so vast, it is only possible to touch lightly and incompletely on the environmental topics in this book. It will be seen that, in comparison with unemployment, housing and poverty, scientific work on our understanding of the impact of environmental changes on human health is only just beginning.

This chapter will touch on a few highlights of general environmental issues, namely global concerns, transport and aesthetic.

## SEVEN ENGINES OF ENVIRONMENTAL DESTRUCTION

There are seven prime engines of destruction: three depletions and four excesses:

1  depletion of finite resources
2  depletion of sustainable resources
3  depletion of the ozone shield
4  excessive heat retention
5  excessive population
6  excessive toxins
7  excessive militarism.

Of these, only those aspects with an immediate impact on health will be mentioned.

## Depletion of finite resources

Depletion of finite or capital resources – coal, oil, gas, minerals and uranium – is a problem that is intrinsic to the nature of the resource. Fritz Schumacher, the renowned guru of the ecological movement, dealt with this matter[1] by stating that the wealth generated from their use should be used to make our economies independent of their further extraction. The depletion itself will lead to shortages and resource wars in the future, unless we act upon Schumacher's advice and transfer our dependence to renewable resources – a scenario that is as realistic as infinite dependence on finite resources is unrealistic.

## Depletion of sustainable resources

It is one thing to wear down a finite or capital resource, but depletion of resources that are in theory infinitely sustainable is another matter entirely. This is clearly an irrational process, like killing the goose that laid the golden egg. The fact that it is occurring throughout the world at an alarming rate demonstrates just how far we are as a species from deserving the self-awarded title of *Homo sapiens*. The loss of renewable resources such as forests (1.3 acres of rainforest are destroyed every second, or 39 million per year) is so well known and discussed that it will not be mentioned here except to mourn the loss of potential medicines through the destruction of biodiversity. Soil loss and depletion of fish stocks are much less widely debated, and are therefore discussed here.

### Soil erosion

Even when it was acceptable to discuss environmental matters in the public arena in the late 1980s, soil erosion was rarely mentioned, yet it is among the most serious of all the problems that we will be handing on to our grandchildren. All farming, even organic, causes soil loss, but the rate of loss is 400% greater for conventional/industrial farming methods. It is estimated that the world loses 25 billion tonnes or 7% of its topsoil each year. Inevitably, as time passes, in 100 or 200 years time, the topsoil will be exhausted, crop yields will fall dramatically and widespread famine will result. Global warming, due to increasing temperatures in the American mid-west ('the breadbasket of the world'), will accelerate this process. It is surprising that politicians give lip service to the notion of 'sustainable development', that is meeting the needs of the current generation without compromising the ability of subsequent generations to meet their needs, while steadfastly avoiding the need to move from industrial farming methods towards the more sustainable organic methods.

## Depletion of fish stocks

Of all the examples of unthinking human greed, the depletion of fish stocks is the most glaringly tragic. This longstanding problem has been a non-issue until the spring 1995 conflict between the Canadians (themselves no innocents in the matter of overfishing) and the Spanish over the residue of the once great fish stocks of the Grand Banks. The North Sea is a fertile source of fish far in excess of its size, because of its relative shallowness. Figure 7.1 shows the steady decline both of the fish catch in the North Sea and, more worryingly, statistical estimates of the remaining stocks of uncaught fish. In some areas cod and haddock are in the 'commercially extinct' category. Pollution of the sea with sewage, which causes over-

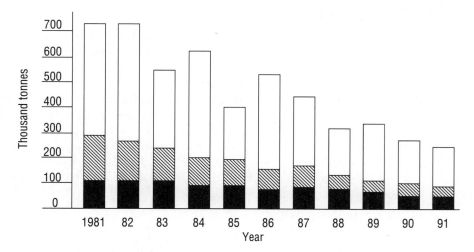

**Figure 7.1** UK and international catches of cod as a proportion of the total stock, thousand tonnes. ■ UK North Sea catch; ▨ remaining international catch; □ uncaught North Sea catch. Reproduced with permission from *The Guardian.*

growths of toxic algae, and chemicals from sources such as chemical weapons and a wide variety of industrial effluents, undoubtedly plays a part in this decline, but the main culprit must be the sheer mindless overfishing that is permitted. Industrial fishing takes half of the North Sea catch for fertilizer or oil. The irony is that fertilizer would not be needed if the sewage were to be treated and returned to the land.

The first, simplest and most easily enforceable control is on net size. Setting a minimum hole size allows immature fish to escape, grow and breed. Even this simple measure is not adhered to. Other measures are setting and enforcing strict quotas and declaring certain areas off-limits for fishing, to allow stocks to recover. The government has tried to restrict the number of days on which a boat can operate. This is not in accord with the need for fishing boats to go with the tide and the weather. A further measure that is not even on the table is restricting the overall size of ships that are allowed to fish, so eliminating the huge factory fishers.

The tragedy is that the threatened loss of fish as an item of diet comes at the same time as we are learning of the great health value of fish as a food. A study in The Netherlands showed that people who ate fish regularly had only half the risk of dying from coronary heart disease of those who did not.[2] Compared with meat, it has a huge advantage in terms of unsaturated and essential fatty acid content, so that if governments do not agree soon to take action to allow stocks to recover, we will lose an opportunity to reduce coronary heart disease. To quantify this loss, let us take a figure of 1% of the 1991 cost of coronary heart disease to the NHS which was £2 720 000 000 as the estimated future annual cost of loss of fish as a healthy item of diet.[3] Thus, the cost to the NHS of loss of fish stocks is £272 million.

## Species/biodiversity loss

An American Indian said that without the animals mankind would die from great loneliness of spirit. Recent estimates are that one species is being lost every 30 minutes. There are 9000 species of birds worldwide. One thousand of these are at risk of extinction, and 6300 species are in decline.[4]

Worse, the world's forests are shrinking at an accelerating rate, and with them the vast wealth of natural medicines that they harbour. We are only just beginning to tap the wealth of plant medicines which are known to the medical wisdom of indigenous tribal healers. Most of the healers, and more of the medicinal herbs, have been wiped out already. Plant extracts have recently been discovered, for instance, that are effective against malaria and AIDS. The cost of this to future medicine has been calculated on the following basis:

1   47 drugs in current use are derived from plants
2   from our knowledge of plant species, and the numbers of species that have yet to be examined for drugs, there should be a further 328 drugs to be found
3   half of all known plant species are to be found in the rainforests
4   from the value of a drug, it can be calculated that the value of drugs in the rainforest is $147 billion.[5]

The cost of discovering these drugs could be reduced if pharmacologists had the humility to listen to native healers instead of mechanistically ploughing through species at random.

In order to derive a cost to the NHS of the loss of rainforest medicines, let us take a figure of 1% of the net ingredient cost of prescriptions. The annual net ingredient cost was £2593 million in 1991, so the loss of future medicines from the rainforest can be valued at £26 million.

## Ozone layer depletion

Much confusion exists in the mind of the populace concerning the twin problems of ozone layer thinning and the greenhouse effect, partly because both occur above our heads, and partly because chlorofluorocarbons (CFCs) are involved in both. Chlorofluorocarbons have three vices: they are extremely longlived, each molecule staying in the atmosphere for 100 years or more (this means that keeping the bathroom window closed while spraying your armpit is of no avail); they are efficient greenhouse gases, trapping solar heat many times more effectively than carbon dioxide; and they are the chief villains in the destruction of the protective stratospheric ozone layer.

Depletion of the ozone layer allows more ultraviolet-B (UV-B) radiation to reach the surface of the Earth. We know that the ozone layer is thinning, but we do not know by exactly how much the UV-B has increased because we have only just begun to measure it in the UK.[6] A report from the Royal Netherlands Meteorological Institute[7] shows how the progressive thinning of the ozone layer is reflected in an increasing amount of UV light reaching the Earth's surface. It may be that some of the variation could be due to sunspot activity or stratospheric dust, but the fact remains that the levels of UV have been shown to be increasing by 10% in one year (Figure 7.2).

We do know however that the incidence of skin cancer, both the common and easily-treated basal cell type and the more serious melanoma type, is increasing in the UK, and that the increase is unlikely to be due to increased sun-bathing alone. It has been estimated that, by the year 2000, 1% of American citizens will have malignant melanoma.

As well as causing these cancers, UV-B also causes sunburn, keratitis (a form of eye irritation), cataracts and a depression of immune functioning certainly in the skin and possibly generally. This immune suppression may be one of the causes of increased skin cancers, as the action of lymphocytes in killing new cancers becomes less effective. The possibility that increased UV-B may affect the immune system generally has been put forward.[8] Non-Hodgkin's lymphomas are a collection of cancers of the lymphocyte-producing tissues, representing about 4% of all cancers. Their incidence has increased over the past few decades with an annual increase of 2–4% observed in Denmark and Sweden. It has been found that non-Hodgkin's lymphoma and skin cancers are strongly correlated, supporting the hypothesis that the increase in UV light may have contributed to the increasing incidence of non-Hodgkin's lymphoma.[9]

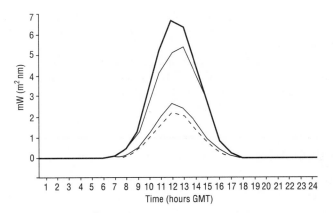

**Figure 7.2** Measurements of UV-B intensity as a function of the hour of the day. *From top to bottom*: the maximum value for February 1993, the maximum value for February 1992, the mean value for February 1993 and the mean value for February 1992. Source: KNMI.

## Cost of ozone depletion

A 5% decrease in the ozone layer is calculated to increase the incidence of UV-B at the Earth's surface by 10%. For every 1% increase in UV-B, a 2% increase in non-melanocytic skin cancer is expected.[10] Taking the 10% per year for northern Europe quoted above, we would expect a 20% increase in skin cancer. It would not be unreasonable therefore to estimate a 0.1–1% increase in the skin disease budget as a result of the ozone layer destruction.

The cost of skin disease to the NHS in 1991 was estimated at £499 million.

|  |  |  |
|---|---|---|
| Cost to the NHS assuming a 0.1% increase due to UV-B | = | £0.5 million |
| Cost to the NHS assuming a 1% increase due to UV-B | = | £5.0 million |

The cost of eye disease to the NHS in 1991 was estimated at £232 million.

|  |  |  |
|---|---|---|
| Cost to the NHS assuming a 0.1% increase due to UV-B | = | £0.2 million |
| Cost to the NHS assuming a 1% increase due to UV-B | = | £2.0 million |
| Estimated annual cost of UV-B caused illness to NHS | = | £7.7 million |

The cost of non-Hodgkin's lymphoma has not been counted.

Health promotion advice centres on modifying citizen's behaviour, that is avoiding sunlight and using high protection factor creams. However, avoiding sunlight itself may have adverse effects, since sunlight creates vitamin D in the skin. Moreover, we are in the process of losing a precious fundamental liberty of enjoying the outdoor life. The magnitude of this loss has not yet entered the consciousness of the average citizen.

# Excessive heat retention: climate change

Computer modelling of global warming (that is the heat-trapping effects of some gases generated by human activity) has become more accurate since the effects of acid aerosols have been included in calculations. It seems that each year brings more weather events that are only expected once in a 100 years or more. In the last 100 years average temperatures have increased by between 0.3 and 0.6°C. The 1980s was the warmest decade on record. The Antarctic ice cap is observed to be receding. Quietly, piece by piece, it seems that the jigsaw is being completed. Global warming, while it still remains a hypothesis subject to more testing, is gaining acceptance as the best available explanation for what is happening to the planet's atmosphere. Attempts by certain extreme right-wing politicians and journalists to 'rubbish' global warming theory have become subdued since their peak in the late '80s. For all practical purposes, we had best assume that global warming is a reality that is happening now and which we must plan for in the future.

The main impact of climate change on health will be through effects on food production and on certain communicable diseases.

## Communicable (infectious) diseases

These diseases are often carried by 'vectors' – rodents or insects. Entomologists can predict where the vectors may be found from isotherms – lines joining areas with the same temperature. Global warming will extend the range of these isotherms, and when Britain is included in an isotherm that allows the vector of an illness to survive we can expect the disease to appear here, at least from time to time.

The *Anopheles* mosquito is a vector for malaria and, depending on the degree of warming, it will be able to survive longer in Britain. More than one out of five planes arriving in Britain has been found to be carrying live mosquitoes, and cases of malaria have occurred in people who have never been abroad, but who live near airports.

Other vector-borne diseases that are liable to occur in a warmer Britain are schistosomiasis, lymphatic filariasis, African trypanosomiasis, leishmaniasis, rickettsiosis, and a few others. Bubonic plague is carried by the rat flea. We are fortunate in that the flea which rides our local brown rat rarely bites humans, but outbreaks of plague in Suffolk in the early years of this century show that it is not impossible for plague to recur. Despite antibiotic treatment, fatality rates for plague stand at 60%.

### Recommendation

That a national effort be made to curb the increase in the rat population and clean up the environmental conditions that allow it to thrive.

## Asthma

If climate change means higher relative humidity in our houses in winter, house dust mite populations will rise, and with them asthma, rhinitis and eczema.

Climate change itself will involve the NHS in greater expenditure on investigation and treatment of tropical diseases. No firm estimates can yet be given of the impact of this on the NHS budget.

## Cockroaches and flies

These may increase in numbers as summer temperatures rise. The effect will be to increase the amount of food-borne disease. Salmonellosis has been estimated to cost the NHS £235 659 per year.[11] If we estimate a 5% increase in these costs due to warming, the extra cost to the NHS will be £11 783 per year. The overall cost to the state was estimated to be £996 399 per year, so a 5% rise, excluding the NHS costs, would come to £38 037 per year out of state spending.

*Shigella sonnei* dysentery has been estimated to cost the state £1 175 289 per year. A 5% increase would add £58 764 to this per year.

## Water-borne disease

Dr Leaf of the Department of Preventative Medicine, Harvard Medical School, has said:[12]

> the condition of water supplies ... is likely to deteriorate further [with climate change]: the intrusion of salt into surface waters as sea levels rise, increased flooding, and runoffs contaminated with pesticides, salts, garbage, excreta, sewage and eroded soil are all likely.

Since 1977 there have been more than 5000 individual cases of disease caused by contaminated drinking water supplies.[13] These can be expected to rise, as can diseases caught through recreational water use. People will also come into contact with sewage in incidents of flooding due to global warming. Finally, storms will cause an increase in injuries due to accidents.

Let us allocate an estimated increased cost to the NHS of £50 000 for these changes.[a]

# Population

Population campaigners have a saying, 'whatever your cause, without stabilizing population, it is a lost cause'. The human population of Earth is rising exponentially (Figure 7.3).

---

[a] For a more detailed look at these problems, see *Potential Impacts of Climate Change on Health in the UK.*[14]

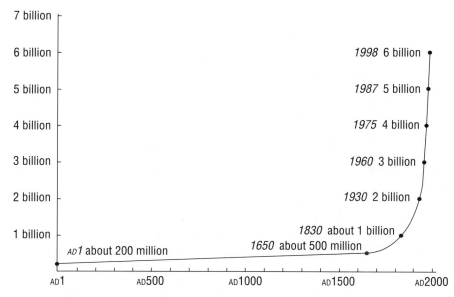

**Figure 7.3** World population trend, AD 1 to AD 2000. Source: Population Concern.

The stabilization of population is an extremely emotive and controversial issue, because of the perceived limitation on the personal liberty to reproduce. However, the sober fact is that we are a biological species, and the growth of all species, from bacteria to humans, is limited by three things:

1  the spatial extent of its habitat
2  the availability of its nutrients
3  the self-inhibiting effect of the toxins it produces.

Ecologists summarize this by speaking of the 'carrying capacity' of the habitat for a given species. In the UK we are exceeding the carrying capacity of our land since we produce less than 50% of the food that we consume. The rest comes to us from imports, often from countries which have difficulty in feeding their own people. If these countries repudiate the debt that forces them to export food in a fruitless attempt to service the debt, we could find ourselves in a food crisis. Our capacity to increase production is severely limited, since we are already operating at or near maximum productivity, and in fact the methods of farming are causing soil erosion that will compromise the ability of our descendants to grow food at the rate that we are achieving. There is no reasonable doubt that starvation in the UK is possibly on the future agenda if we continue to ignore this problem.

The question is not therefore, 'Need we limit population growth?' but 'Shall we limit population growth now through education and voluntary consent, or will we leave it to future authoritarian governments to limit it through compulsion?'

Population limitation begins at home. There is no point in preaching control to developing countries if we have not achieved limitation in the UK. The population in the UK is at present increasing with an annual growth rate of 0.3%.

If this rate of growth were to continue, in 50 years the population of the UK would increase to 67 371 250 – an increase of 16%. However, it has been argued that the current increase is the result of growth in previous years, so that although the birth rate is presently below replacement level population growth is expected to continue for 30 years.[15] Fertility has a kind of momentum since each woman is fertile for 30 years. Therefore the postwar 'bulge' of population will produce another 'sub-bulge' of children even though their fertility is less than the previous generation. For the generation born after 1950 the family size is below the level of replacement, so that the population level is expected to begin to fall in the UK after the year 2007.

It is difficult to determine the effect of social class on fertility rates since it is almost impossible to place women accurately into social classes.[16] Using the area method of classification, and using unemployment as a crude measure of deprivation, there is a suggestion that unemployment by region is associated with increased fertility, especially among women under 20 (Figure 6.2). Northern Ireland falls outside the trend, with a lower birth rate for the under-20s. If further research does confirm that fertility is greater among the deprived, one cause may be that if a person's life is restricted and grey because of material deprivation, the perfection, love and joy that a baby brings may be a powerful motive to bring one into the world. In view of the chaos, stress and hassle that the subsequent toddler imports into life, this decision may be seen as irrational, but irrationality is a basic part of the human condition.

The issue of young single mothers has been the focus of much political debate recently, and indeed there has been a marked rise in the number of babies born outside marriage (Figure 7.4). International comparisons for live births outside marriage show the UK with less than Sweden, Denmark and France, on a par with the USA, and ahead of the rest of the EU countries.

Many GPs have a distinct impression that the main cause for pregnancy among some single young women is not so much a great desire to jump the queue for council housing as a common or garden loss of inhibitions as a result of getting drunk at a party. Pregnant schoolgirls who come for abortion counselling have been questioned about their knowledge of the facts of life. Their knowledge is fine, but they confess that it seemed irrelevant at the time, because they were drunk.

## Recommendation

That sex education lessons should contain warnings that excess alcohol can lead to unwanted increase in abdominal girth.

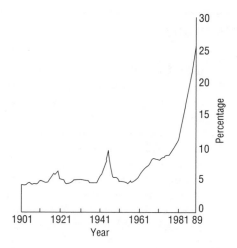

**Figure 7.4**  Livebirths outside marriage. Source: Office of Population Censuses and Surveys, General Register Office (Scotland) 1991.

Another factor in the increase in single-parent families is thought to be that young men no longer have a defined role as the breadwinner. When income is in benefits, and in some cases, such as mortgage interest income support, conditional upon being out of work, the man may be seen as a noisy and troublesome encumbrance, useful only for fertilization purposes.

The social and environmental conditions that encourage these trends must be altered if we are to cap our population growth and so set an example to the rest of the world.

## The ageing population

One aspect that must be mentioned is the increasing age of the population. The numbers of people aged 75 or over increased by 50% between the 1981 and 1991 censuses. If this trend continues, the proportion of able-bodied people to care for the elderly, or to earn taxable wealth to pay for their care, will be low. This is a problem if employment is seen as an economic cost to be borne by the state, rather than as an opportunity to give meaningful work to people who would otherwise be unemployed.

The costs to the NHS through overcrowding and future shortages of food are incalculable. Let us assign to them a notional value of 0.1% of the 1991 NHS budget, rounded down to £31 000 million.

## Excessive toxins

This topic will be covered in chapter 8.

# Nuclear proliferation and militarism

It is established that global nuclear war would overwhelm the medical services of the 'civilized' world that introduced these weapons. Although it would be possible theoretically to save some of the lives of the injured who were admitted to treatment through a strict triage system, in practice there would be an unprecedented demand for medical services, which would be in very short supply. Not only would there be a loss of medical personnel through death, illness or desire to be with their families, but there would also be a lack of production and distribution of the antibiotics, fluid replacement and administration sets, not to mention operative equipment, needed to help. Therefore prevention is the only solution.

Nuclear deterrence is presented as the way of preventing nuclear war. Deterrence is a complex web of technological and human control systems that is anything but infallible. During the Cold War, nuclear strategists said that we could not disarm while communism existed. Now that communism no longer exists, it has suddenly been discovered that the Islamic bomb is the real threat. Chaotic lack of international controls on the strategic arsenals of the old USSR means that plutonium is leaking across borders to these countries, almost as if to fulfil the prophecy. Britain, France and the USSR aided Iraq's efforts to obtain the bomb.[17] The Nuclear Non-Proliferation Treaty (NPT) is in disrepute because within days of its renewal in 1995 China and France cynically restarted tests. Non-nuclear nations justifiably object to the fact that nuclear nations have not honoured their side of the NPT agreement by limiting their own arsenals and ceasing to carry out tests.

The attitude of denial cannot exist forever. Once serious questions are asked regarding the fallibility of the deterrence system, and the costs of the deterrent itself, political and public opinion will force Britain to join the vast majority of psychologically mature nations that do not feel the need to threaten the world with destruction in order to feel secure.

The financial benefits of this transaction are impressive. The capital costs of the Trident submarines – £12 billion – are lost forever, but the running costs are there to be saved. The government admits that it costs £125 000 per hour to keep Trident afloat, and Greenpeace's estimates for this figure are £195 000. A large proportion of this amount of taxpayers' money can be diverted into constructive and rational projects when Trident is withdrawn and decommissioned. Let us assume that £500 million per year would be available for the NHS if Trident were to be scrapped.

Militarism itself – the mindset that believes that security can be created through making another party feel deeply insecure – is a drain on the economy, despite the fact that the UK is the world's fourth largest arms producer. The phenomenal economic success of Japan and Germany since the Second World War is in no small part related to the fact that they were disarmed. Deprived of the need to maintain armies, navies and airforce, and denied the opportunity to manufacture weaponry, the defeated powers were forced to turn their hands to making goods that people actually use in their everyday lives, such as cars, radios and refrigerators.

The result was that they overtook countries whose economies were burdened and distorted with the trappings of militarism.

The truth is that the world cannot afford generals. The real enemy is not other states but the state of the world. Our future is insecure not because communism may rise again and come to strangle us in our beds, or because mad Mullahs may take over Whitehall, but because the stability of the natural and social environment on which we depend is compromised. It is possible to rectify the damage and to create a system that is compatible with our long-term survival and health, but only if all our energies and resources are put into the task. Militarism is an expensive diversion from the historic task that our generation faces.

Militarism must be expressed as opportunity costs and the increased risk of war. Let us count it conservatively as 0.1% of the 1991 NHS budget, that is £30 million.

These then are the major, global environmental threats that we must face up to. While taking the broad view, we should take in three further overall problems: emergent viral infections, the aesthetic environment and transport.

# NEW VIRAL INFECTIONS

Viruses are tiny particles which are stripped down to the bare essentials that a living organism needs: a core of DNA or RNA wrapped in a protein coat. Their effects range from mild inconvenience to near-certain death.

## Minor viral illnesses

There is a general perception that viral illnesses are becoming more common as time passes. Whereas people used to get perhaps one cold per year, they now feel that they are getting four or five, and that they are characterized by more 'flu-like fever and aching than before. On theoretical grounds, it would be expected that increased travel, both international and within the nation, would be expected to bring about increasing infections, as the more people we meet, the more likely we are to pick up an infection. This expectation is consistent with the Kinlen hypothesis (chapter 11). On a more depressing note, increased susceptibility to viral infection is also consistent with the supposition that our immune systems are becoming incompetent under the burden of chemical challenge, stress and poor diet.

Figures taken from *Morbidity Statistics from General Practice* (OPCS),[18] gathered every ten years from 60 sample practices all over the UK, might suggest an increase in minor respiratory infections. Unfortunately, interpretation of these data is bedevilled by changes in categories for collection each time data were collected. If, however, we assume that acute nasopharyngitis (1955–56), nasopharyngitis (febrile or non-febrile) (1971–72), upper respiratory infection (non-febrile or febrile) (1981–82) and minor disease of the respiratory system (1991–92) are all

**Table 7.2**  Trends in consultations for minor respiratory infections

| Year | Rate per 1000 population |
|------|--------------------------|
| 1955–56 | 81.1 |
| 1971–72 | 96.2 |
| 1980–82 | 170.9 |
| 1991–92 | 195.7 |

Source: *Morbidity Statistics from General Practice* (OPCS).[18]

diagnostic categories referring to roughly the same conditions, a steady increase in consultations is apparent (Table 7.2).

It must be said that records from the author's own practice do not support this impression. In a general practice of 4000 rural patients, the reason for all personal consultations between 1979 and 1981 were recorded manually. Computer records for the two years 1988–90 are available for comparison (Table 7.3).

The absence of 'viral infection' categories in the 1979–81 survey is the result of change in diagnostic labelling, since at that time the ''flu' category was used. Although the composited figures for 'viral infection' and 'influenza and 'flu-like' would show a marked rise, this cannot be interpreted as a rising trend, because it covered a minor outbreak of 'flu-like illness in the later years. The downward trend for the total figures may reflect the steady downward pressure exerted over the years against coming to surgery with minor illness. The message that antibiotics are ineffective against colds may have got through, reflected in the three-fold reduction in coryza consultations. These data do not support, but also do not necessarily refute, the hypothesis that minor viral illnesses are becoming more common.

If further research does confirm that viral illnesses are becoming more common, this would be another health cost to be set down against transportation.

**Table 7.3**  Reasons for personal consultations

| Diagnosis | 1979–81 | 1988–90 |
|-----------|---------|---------|
| Viral infection | 0 | 138 |
| Influenza and 'flu-like | 131 | 185 |
| Cough and bronchitis | 587 | 537 |
| Sinusitis | 197 | 123 |
| Sore throat | 256 | 178 |
| Coryza (i.e. common cold) | 79 | 25 |
| Total | 1250 | 1049 |

# Major viral illnesses

Acquired immunodeficiency syndrome is not the only disease to present humanity with a new threat and health services with new expenses. A variety of emergent viruses are poised to enter the arena, whether through natural mutations or through human interference.

Ebola virus was first identified in an outbreak in Ebola, Zaire, Central Africa. It is a very severe infection, with the following characteristics:

- transmission is by body fluids (except Ebola Reston, which is air transmissible)
- the incubation period is between two and 21 days
- onset is severe, with headache, red eyes, fever, shivering, aching muscles, rash, vomiting and (bloody) diarrhoea
- haemorrhaging occurs internally and through all orifices
- death occurs in between 30% and 88% of cases a few days after onset from general systems failure.

There is no treatment available. The only useful response is for the public to refrain from travelling in order to prevent spread.

Little is known about the natural history of the virus. It may infect monkeys but they are unlikely to be the main reservoir. Recently, suspicion has focused on the occupants, possibly bats, of a cave in northern Zaire. Whatever the reservoir, it is clear that it appears recently to have developed the capability of 'jumping' to humans.

So far four outbreaks have occurred and three different types of virus have been identified:

1976    Ebola Zaire caused 500 deaths
1979    Ebola Sudan
1989    Ebola Reston (Washington DC), a US government monkey laboratory. This strain was transmissible by air, but was harmless to humans
1995    Ebola outbreak in Kikwit, Zaire.

Different strains have emerged with each outbreak. If a strain arrives that is transmissible by air, and also pathogenic to humans, the consequences could be serious. It is not known exactly why the disease has appeared now, and whether there is a connection with the fact that the AIDS virus also emerged from Central Africa. It has been speculated that the Central African rainforest, as a high-rainfall area, received a high dose of radiation from the atmospheric nuclear weapons tests, and that this may have induced mutations in viruses. What is certain is that viral diseases hitch rides on modern methods of transport. The transport of monkeys out of Africa for whatever reason carries great risks, and must be intensively regulated and policed.

## Waste disposal from British Rail trains

Before leaving the subject of infection, the surprising method of disposing excrement from British trains must be mentioned. In 1994, 55% of passenger trains did not have retention tanks but dropped waste directly on the track. When the toilet of a speeding train is flushed, the contents form an aerosol that is taken into the train's air supply and dispersed throughout the train. The knowledge that a train moving at 60 mph has progressed 200 feet during the flushing process is of small comfort for the passengers at the rear of a train longer than 200 feet. The Department of Transport Railways Directorate admits that 'There is a current lack of information regarding train toilet discharge though current research suggests that the risk of contracting disease from it is negligible'. The research quoted was an examination of the risk to people working on the underframe of trains,[19] not passengers exposed to the faecal and urinary aerosol. The Health and Safety Executive is 'not aware of any cases of people becoming ill as a result of toilet discharge from trains.' This reflects the fact that passengers are blissfully ignorant of the fact that they are exposed to vaporized '*eau de toilette*'. Clearly, there is a need for epidemiological studies of the health of passengers who travel on trains with retention tanks compared with that of passengers who travel on those fitted with the aerosol option. We can be confident that, with privatization, the new companies will be more than happy to carry out this research in the name of customer care. Perhaps.

# AESTHETICS

In Britain, unlike on the Continent of Europe, the word 'aesthetic' is not in common use. The substitute words that we use leave an uncovered gap: 'pretty' is associated with inconsequential qualities and 'beautiful' indicates an extreme, not commonplace, set of qualities, and both have feminine connotations. Yet the 'aesthetic', denoting a set of circumstances which are well coordinated and have a pleasing effect on the perceiver, is of considerable importance to everyday well-being. Depressed persons see the world about them as colourless, ugly and lifeless. Conversely, people living in colourless, ugly and lifeless environments may be expected to become depressed.

Backing for this theory comes from the experience of the charity Learning Through Landscapes, which began in 1989 to encourage schools to tear up asphalt playgrounds and lay down grass and shrubs instead. Many of the 600 participating schools reported that playground misbehaviour and bullying decreased significantly after the greening of the playgrounds.[20]

# The visual environment

A wide-ranging programme to paint, tidy, plant flowers and trees in and otherwise beautify public spaces will certainly create good work, and may reasonably be expected to improve the general morale of the people who live in the new environment, with resultant savings in depression-related illness and a degree of increased productivity.

One important aspect of the degradation of the visual environment is the ubiquitous presence of litter. Not only our cities, but also the countryside are polluted with plastic bags, confectionery wrappings and cigarette packets. The extent of hedgerow littering can only be appreciated by cyclists or pedestrians. The effect is to dull or block the soul-reviving appreciation of the forms of nature with a constant resentful reverie on the thoughtlessness and barbarity of the human species.

The introduction of a £2000 fine for people caught dropping litter, at Mrs Thatcher's personal behest, has not had a marked effect on the amounts of litter in our streets and hedgerows because of the difficulty in getting prosecutions. Concerned citizens who spot people dropping litter are reluctant to intervene because of the possibility of causing an unpleasant scene, and are even less likely to be prepared to witness against them in court, since this is likely to involve one or two days in the legal process. Many might also feel that, however they dislike litter, they would feel less than comfortable with being instrumental in putting another into debt for £2000 over littering. Table 7.4 shows that convictions for littering have more than halved since the 1990 Act brought in the £2000 fine. This change is not compensated by an increase in cautions, since the number of cautions has fallen from 322 in 1992 to 82 in 1993.

Since draconian punishment is not effective, prevention and cleaning are therefore the only options available. The 'polluter pays' principle can usefully be applied to cover the costs of cleaning. Most litter consists of confectionery and cigarette wrappers. It is impossible to catch the perpetrator, but it is possible to apply a levy on each packet of confectionery and tobacco sold. The proceeds of this levy would be passed to local authorities for the purpose of paying for cleaning up litter. An additional option is to require that packaging of the sort that commonly ends up as litter should be made of biodegradable materials only.

In addition to the aesthetics, there is an economically beneficial aspect to removing litter. Sheets of plastic become air-borne in high winds, and some will become entangled in telephone and electricity wires, increasing their aerodynamic drag to the point that some wires are brought down. A thorough eradication of litter will therefore reduce repair costs following gales to some extent.

**Table 7.4** Convictions for littering

| Year | No. of convictions |
| --- | --- |
| 1989 | 2174 |
| 1990 | 2212 |
| 1991 | 1397 |
| 1992 | 1344 |
| 1993 | 988 |

Source: Home Office, personal communication.

The costs of litter eradication can be seen as an investment rather than a recurring outlay. Public consciousness will be raised when people note with pleasure that their environment has made a change for the better, and people who would not think about adding to an already littered environment may be inhibited from throwing the first piece into a pristine space.

If these industries are required to pay for the litter that they generate, this would not only remedy the assault on the visual environment that they generate, but would also bring downward pressure on the consumption of their products and, third, motivate these industries to use their considerable advertising influence to raise public awareness against littering.

## Recommendation

That a levy should be place on all confectionery, tobacco and plastic products and set at such a level that when diverted to local authorities it is sufficient to pay for a countrywide litter-picking operation.

# TRANSPORT

Between 1950 and 1990 the world population increased by 15%; over the same time period the number of cars increased by 1000%.

- Between 40 and 80 per cent of major pollutants come from motor cars.
- Twenty per cent of carbon dioxide and CFC emissions emanate from cars.
- In the USA, roads, parking lots, etc. have consumed 10% of all arable land.

Transport policy in the UK is heavily biased in favour of the motor car. The Department of Transport proudly placards its road-building efforts as 'Investing in Roads', whereas the railways are denied realistic investment and criticized if they do not make a profit. The motorist pays £14–15 billion in road fund licence, but this is at a conservative estimate only 41% of the full cost of motoring. Other estimates[21] suggest that the motorist pays only 27% of the full cost.

The Royal Commission on Environmental Pollution (RCEP) Report on Transport[22] estimated that road transport costs in the UK come to at least £10–18.3 billion, of which £5.4 billion is ascribed to traffic accidents (Table 7.5). A constant 1% of GNP of any country in the world is lost in road traffic accidents. For incomprehensible reasons, a human life is costed at £800 000 if lost on roads but £3 million if lost on railways.

Unquantifiable costs of motoring are:

- loss of land and access to land

- visual intrusion
- severance of communities (that is inability of people easily to meet with each other across the road)
- loss of habitats
- costs of air pollution on human health
- costs of air pollution on environment.

The motorist is therefore getting a free ride on the back of the taxpayer, 50% of whom have no access to a car. The Royal Commission sought to achieve a balance between the needs of the motorist and the needs of the rest of mankind: another view is that, in the interests of balance, non-motorized transport should be given priority.

**Table 7.5**  Costs of motoring

| Item costed | Cost (£ million) |
| --- | --- |
| Congestion | 15 000 |
| Roads | |
|    Capital expenditure | 3 650 |
|    Repairs and maintenance | 2 153 |
|    Cleaning | 100 |
|    Administration | 146 |
|    Research, design, safety | 32 |
| Deaths and injuries | 4 803 |
| Policing | 400 |
| Licensing costs | 150 |
| Company car subsidy | 2 400 |
| Pollution | |
|    Air | 2 500 |
|    Global warming | 657 |
|    Noise | 2 100 |
| Total cost of motoring | 34 091 |

Source: *Costing the Benefits: the Value of Cycling* (Cyclists' Touring Club).[23]

The Royal Commission Report set out 110 recommendations, which should be taken whole, not piecemeal. A few selected recommendations are as follows.

1  In planning for new roads, the first step should be to query the need for them: the planning priority should be to minimize the need for transportation.
2  The motor car should be controlled both by regulation and by fiscal means: fuel duty, road pricing, parking charges. Public transport should be supported.
3  Cycleways must be developed wholesale; bits and pieces which lead from nowhere to nowhere do not get used.
4  Pedestrianization must be developed.
5  Public transport needs passenger-friendly stations, and must be convenient, reliable, cheap and 'seamlessly connected'. ('Integrated' is not a politically correct word in UK government circles in the 1990s.)

6 Measures to discourage car use may have synergistic effects. Measures A, B and C might each produce a 3% reduction in car use, but applied together they might produce a 20% reduction. Wholesale commitment is required.
7 Overall speed restriction should be introduced.
8 Road freight could be reduced by:
   - increasing the cost of road freight
   - restricting passage through cities
   - investing in rail freight.

It is apparent from this that the arguments for a radical realignment of transport policy away from the motor car are so strong that even a Royal Commission can be swayed by them.

## The case for cycling[a]

The health gains from exercise are well known, affecting incidence of:

- cardiovascular heart disease
- stroke
- osteoporosis
- diabetes mellitus
- cancer
- loss of muscle mass
- stress-related illness
- death (exercise contributes to longevity).

Structured exercise (sport, workouts, swimming, etc.) needs motivation, persistence, self-discipline, time and money. Many couch potatoes turn over a new leaf with resolve to take regular exercise, follow it enthusiastically for two or three weeks, only to fall by the wayside when the new routine is interrupted by a holiday or cold weather. It is unrealistic to expect the nation to benefit from swimming when there is only one pool to 46 000 people in the UK.

Cycling and brisk walking solve these problems as they are tied in to the daily pattern of living. Seventy-five per cent of journeys are under five miles. These could be replaced by cycling or walking.

## Making way for the cycle

The problem is that we are in a vicious circle. Even people who would prefer to cycle are deterred by the perceived danger to their safety posed by heavy traffic and the health risk of breathing large quantities of polluted air. They therefore use their car to take their children to school or to the shops, which makes the pollu-

[a] I am indebted to Dr Mayer Hillman, Senior Fellow Emeritus at Policy Studies Institute for much of the material in this section.

tion worse. Exhortation is not enough: public policies have to change to provide incentives and a safe environment for cyclists, to provide frequent, cheap and clean public transport, and to put steady downward pressure on car use by withdrawing the 60% subsidy that the motorist presently enjoys.

Although there is a 1:25 000 000 risk of a cyclist being killed on the roads, the risk of not cycling through life years lost from the conditions listed above is greater: the ratio of life years gained through extra fitness to life years lost through accidents is 20:1.[24] This ratio can be increased by making cycling safer through cycleways.

The targets for cycleways set by the RCEP Transport and the Environment report are modest in the extreme, aiming for only 10% of journeys in ten years. This target is only one-third of current use in The Netherlands. If the plan by Sustrans[25] is adopted by the Millennium Fund, a 5000-mile cycleway by the year 2000 could become a reality. In September 1995 Sustrans was allocated £43 million. This grant can be set in perspective by noting that the Department of Transport is prepared to spend at least £11 million on widening one mile of the M4 motorway near Portishead without considering the low-cost option of traffic flow management which would make the widening unnecessary.

## Costings

Figure 7.5 gives a comparison of the amount of cycleway provided in The Netherlands and Denmark compared with the UK, and Figure 7.6 compares the cycleway provision in Bristol and Hannover. The Continentals have far to go on their bikes, whereas we have far to go in our conceptualization planning and development. The cycleways must be well planned and constructed, otherwise they will not be used or will be dangerous in use. Each kilometre costs between £40 000 and £50 000 to construct, although these costs would be less if some of the labour benefited from the wage subsidy. Cycle lanes painted on roads cost £12 000 per kilometre.

The cost of a 1200-km cycle network for London is the same as 400 yards of new underground line. One mile of motorway costs as much as 5000 miles of cycleway. Cycleways are 100–600 times cheaper than Urban Light Railway.

A report[23] for the Cyclists' Touring Club estimates that the economy would be £1.3 billion better off if 20% of journeys were made by bike, and £4.6 billion better off if 50% of journeys were to be made by bike. The 20% figure is feasible with minimum change, since 75% of car journeys are under five miles, 50% are under two miles and 32% are under a mile.

## Protecting the pedestrian

Cycleways and lanes provide a relatively safe haven for cyclists. Pedestrians also need this shelter. The Dutch have given the name '*Woonerf*' or living space to protected areas of towns where the child has right of way and motor cars are severely restricted.

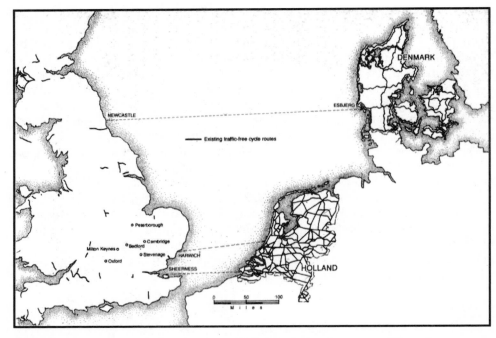

**Figure 7.5** European national cycle routes. This map shows the extent of long-distance cycle routes in various European countries. These are signposted and named inter-regional routes connecting town and country and utilizing purpose-made cycle paths and quiet, safe by-roads. In The Netherlands alone these routes combine to form a complete network of about 6000 km with connections to ferry services and routes abroad. Guidebooks are widely available in which the routes are clearly described and reproduced on maps. In addition to those shown, there are literally thousands of kilometres more of recommended cycle routes, primarily using roads with very low volumes of motor traffic, but using especially constructed facilities wherever necessary. *Solid line*: existing long-distance national cycle routes. Source: Sustrans.

## Journeys

New planning polices are being introduced which are designed to reduce the amount of travelling that people have to do. It must be said that these policies appeared in the Green Party's *Manifesto for a Sustainable Society* in the early 1970s.

Social journeys to visit family and friends account for 26% of total. At least some of these journeys must reflect the social dislocation caused by the business policy known as 'spiralling'. Promotion in a business is usually to a branch of the organization in a different part of the country. The breadwinner is obliged to move and the family is uprooted to follow the job. This poses considerable strains on the family. First there is often a period, which can go on for many months, when the breadwinner and family are separated while the home is sold. Next, old friendships of all the family are disrupted, which is especially painful for children. Finally, much

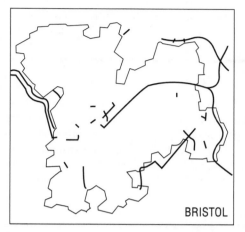 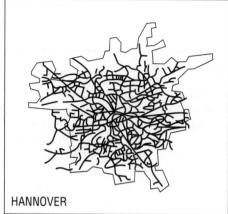

BRISTOL | HANNOVER

**Figure 7.6** Cycleways comparison – Bristol, UK, and Hannover, Germany. *Solid lines:* traffic-free routes, separate cycleways or shared-use footways. Traffic lanes on highways, special crossings and advisory routes are not shown. Source: Sustrans.

travelling is entailed in visiting old friends and families. These costs should be borne in mind by businesses when endorsing spiralling as an occupational policy.

Home working or tele-cottaging, in which workers work from home, using computer links and communications, may help to diminish journey times in the long run, although it carries with it the same problem as unemployment, that is the loss of beneficial and stimulating social links with colleagues.

## Limiting traffic speed

One of the most effective measures to curb the car is a 55 mph overall speed limit universally, and 20 mph in built-up areas. The 55 mph limit is already in place in the USA, and is universally respected. Speed limitation decreases pollution and fuel consumption, decreases the frequency and severity of accidents and gives a competitive advantage to railways, which will offer shorter journey times. Fuel efficiency is optimized at 50 mph, and nitrogen oxide emissions are less at 50 than at 80 mph. In towns, 20 mph limits would not only reduce the severity of accidents (Table 7.6), but would also, paradoxically, improve the flow of traffic in towns. Traffic that accelerates up to 35 mph in clear patches and

**Table 7.6** Effect of speed on child deaths in accidents

| Impact speed (mph) | Children killed (%) |
| --- | --- |
| 40 | 85 |
| 20 | 5 |

then brakes at a congested patch makes slower progress than traffic that flows at a steady 20 mph.

## Signage

One very simple and low-cost measure to decrease traffic flow in towns is to invest in better signage. Anyone who has experienced the frustration of getting lost and driving fruitlessly in circles looking for parking facilities or other destinations will agree that better signs would cut this pointless driving. Out-of-town consultants would be needed to assess and advise the local transport authority, since local officers, already familiar with the layout of the town, are less conscious of the need for clear signs.

## Gross polluters

Traffic pollution is not evenly spread. Sixty per cent of cars (the cleaner set) produce only 9% of the total traffic-generated carbon monoxide pollution, while the dirtiest 12% of cars produce 50% of the total carbon monoxide. Clearly, these 'gross polluters' should be targeted, and at present there are two approaches which are being tested. One is to have random tests at roadside points, manned by police and environmental health officers (EHOs). This is a labour-intensive operation, and neither the police nor the environmental health departments can easily afford to tie their officers up in this way. The second alternative on offer is to use technology that instantly analyses emissions of passing cars and photographs the number plates of offenders who exceed the limits. The drawback to this elegant technological solution is the capital cost and vulnerability of the equipment. A third, equally elegant, but very low cost, solution is to require that all heavy goods vehicles display the number of the Dirty Diesel reporting telephone line. This has two immediate effects: first, it publicizes the existence of the line, so that more concerned citizens will be aware of its existence, and second, it ensures that all vehicles bearing the number will be optimally tuned and clean, since no sane fleet manager is going to send out a smoky vehicle with the report line emblazoned on the back. Gross polluters are in the end totally unnecessary, since they are a sign of a badly tuned and therefore inefficient engine. Economic costs cannot in this case be used to defend against environmental improvements.

## Road pricing

This is a possible method of compelling motorists to pay for roads. Large toll areas can be avoided by using high-technology sensors to pick up signals from cars using the roads and bill the car owner automatically. The disadvantage is twofold:

the high capital cost of installing the equipment and the effect it will have in excluding the poor from using the roads.

# REFERENCES

1    Schumacher F (1973) *Small is Beautiful*. Abacus, London.

2    Kromhout D, Feskens E J, Bowles C H (1995) The protective effect of a small amount of fish on coronary heart disease mortality in an elderly population. *Int J Epidemiol*: **24(2)**; 340–5.

3    Chew R (1992) *Compendium of Health Statistics (8th edn)*. Office of Health Economics, London. Sect. 83.

4    Brown L R, Flavin C, Kane H (1993) *Vital Signs. Worldwatch 1992/1993*. Earthscan, London.

5    Mendelsohn R and Balick M J (1995) The value of undiscovered pharmaceuticals. *Economic Botany*: **49(2)**; 223–8.

6    Driscoll C M H, Whillock M J, Dean S F (1992) *Solar Radiation Measurements at Three Sites in the UK May 1990–April 1991*. National Radiological Protection Board NRPB–M344, Didcot.

7    van Zijst P (1993) Thinner ozone layer leads to more UV radiation. *Change*: **16**; 1.

8    Kripke M L (1981) Immunologic mechanisms in UV radiation carcinogenesis. *Adv Cancer Res*: **34**; 69–106.

9    Adami J, Frish M, Yuen J *et al.* (1995) Evidence of an association between non-Hodgkin's lymphoma and skin cancer. *BMJ*: **310**; 1491–5.

10   Australian Environment Council (1987) *Environmental, Health and Economic Implications of the use of Chlorofluorocarbons as Aerosol Propellants and Possible Substitutes*. Australian Government Publishing Service, Canberra.

11   Sockett P N and Roberts J A (1991) The social and economic impact of salmonellosis. *Epidemiol Infect*: **107**; 335–47.

12   Leaf A (1989) Potential health effects of global climatic change and environmental changes. *N Eng J Med*: **321**; 1577–83.

13   Galbraith N S, Barrett N J, Stanwell-Smith R (1987) Water and disease after Croydon: a review of water-borne and water-associated disease in the UK 1937–1986. *J Inst Water Environ Management*: **1**; 7–20.

14   Greenpeace (1994) *Potential Impacts of Climate Change on Health in the UK*. Greenpeace, London.

15   Craig J (1994) Replacement level fertility and future population growth. *Popul Trends*: **78**; 20–2.

16   Botting B and Cooper J (1994) Analysing fertility and infant mortality by mother's class as defined by occupation. *Pop Trends*: **78**; 20–2.

17   Lawson R (1995) Nuclear arms for Iraq. *Med War*: **11**; 28–33.

18   OPCS (1993) *Morbidity Statistics from General Practice.* OPCS, London.

19   London School of Hygiene and Tropical Medicine (1991) *Occupational Health Problems Associated with Working on Vehicle Underframes.* LSHTM, London.

20   McIlroy A J (1995) *Daily Telegraph.* May 4. London.

21   Whitelegg J (1992) *Traffic Congestion: Is there a Way Out?* Leading Edge Press and Publishing, Hawes.

22   Royal Commission on Environmental Pollution (1994) *Transport and the Environment, 18th Report.* Cm 2674. HMSO, London.

23   Shayler M, Fergusson M, Rowell A (1993) *Costing the Benefits: the Value of Cycling.* Cyclist's Touring Club, Godalming.

24   Mayer H M (1992) *Cycling and the Promotion of Health.* Proceedings of the PTRC Conference. Policy Studies Institute, London.

25   Sustrans Campaigns for Cycleways in the UK, 35 King Street, Bristol BS1 4DZ.

# 8

# Our strained relations with environmental agents

*Only within the moment of time represented by this present century has one
species – man – acquired significant power to alter the nature of his world.*

Rachel Carson[1]

## INTRODUCTION

We are surrounded by, and constantly interacting with, environmental agents that
may affect the well-being of our physical self for good or ill. Although the number
of agents is seemingly endless, there are a limited number of effects which environmental agents have on our cells. They may:

1  kill cells outright. Irritants, acids, alkalis and other agents may do this if their
   concentration is sufficiently high. This affects body surfaces and may produce
   reddening and itching of the skin, soreness in the throat and eyes, coughing,
   and in the gut, vomiting or diarrhoea
2  produce an immune system response, resulting either in elimination of the
   antigen or possibly in some kind of an allergic response
3  affect chemistry of the cell, by making it more acidic or alkaline, or by producing 'free radicals'
4  affect the cell's DNA structure, which may result in either imperfect repair or
   production of faulty information. In the latter case, cancer or deformed offspring may be the result
5  mimic the action of the body's messengers and hormones, notably oestrogens
6  affect the nervous system by slowing or stopping nerve activity
7  cause other reactions that are not yet recognized.

## New environmental conditions, new diseases?

Investigations into the effects of environmental agents concentrate on definite events that can be measured without dispute, such as death or cancer. More subtle conditions such as tiredness, apparent depression or general increase in low-grade illness are not picked up by these methods. Viewed in this light, environmental epidemiology is still in its infancy. A prodigious amount of work is necessary to decide each point of scientific debate, and it is entirely possible that we are missing a large amount of environmentally induced illness through not rightly knowing what to look for. The effects of tobacco would not have been recognized without the presence of a comparative group of non-smokers – yet where is the comparable population that is not affected to some degree by environmental pollution?

Just as an overworked GP may miss the early signs of serious illness in a patient simply because his or her 'index of suspicion' has been lulled into sleep as a result of seeing large numbers of minor conditions, so also we may be unaware of major environmentally induced changes that are taking place under our noses. Environmental concern has in the past been seen by physicians as a field of enquiry separate from medicine. Early concerns and hypotheses about possible effects of environmental agents should rightly be treated with a healthy degree of scientific scepticism: but often the scepticism goes beyond the scientific stance to the more emotive 'pooh-pooh' reaction of denial. This reaction often finds its mirror in the reaction of the proponent of the hypothesis, who may feel personally hurt by the reception given to the discovery, and may begin to counter-attack. Soon the situation arises that if one side says 'white' the other will automatically say 'black'. These unhelpful divides could be averted by proper regard on both sides for the scientific method and for respect for the human needs of those with whom we may not agree.

## SCIENTIFIC METHOD

It is exceedingly difficult to 'prove' that any environmental agent is the cause of a given illness. In fact, science never 'proves' anything in the QED sense of school geometry: the best status that a scientific hypothesis can enjoy is 'not yet disproven'.

In order to try to clarify matters, Dr Bradford Hill put forward a set of criteria to govern the way we decide whether a condition may be caused by an environmental agent. They are not a 'gold standard', but a tarnished and nevertheless useful 'brass standard'.[2]

The Bradford Hill criteria are as follows.

1   Strength. The people exposed to the agent should be very definitely iller than the unaffected population. This tends to overlook the action of agents which make people only slightly ill.

2   Consistency. Different workers should be arriving at the same conclusions. This presupposes the adequate availability of research funds.

3   Specificity. Hill himself admitted that this was not a strong criterion, because nature is rarely so kind to researchers as to determine that, for instance, all mobile telephone users get one particular kind of brain cancer.

4   Temporality. The suspected cause must precede the development of the disease. Uncontroversial.

5   Biological gradient. The greater the exposure to the agent, the greater should be the degree of illness.

6   Plausibility. It is helpful if there is a known biological mechanism to explain the effect. Hill admits this is helpful if it exists, but absence of biological knowledge should not cause us to dismiss a causative relationship. Yet this absence was the sole reason for the Clayton Committee to dismiss the illnesses in the Camelford scandal (see p. 149).

7   Coherence. The causal hypothesis should not seriously conflict with our present knowledge of disease. This is the converse of the plausibility argument, and shares its weakness. Indeed, it is basically unscientific, since it assumes that our present knowledge is correct, whereas in fact our present knowledge should always be judged and revised in the light of new, well-established data.

8   Experiment. Hill says, 'For instance, because of an observed association some preventive action is taken. Does it in fact prevent?' This is an important and positive criterion, yet is an approach that is conspicuous by its absence in the UK.

9   Analogy. For example, past experience with thalidomide will make us more ready to look for an association between drugs in pregnancy and birth deformities.

These are excellent and reasonable criteria, in theory. In practice, it took 20 years of intensive work by many researchers to establish what is now taken as a self-evident fact – that smoking is bad for health. Given that rate of progress for every new environmental agent that arrives (at a rate of 2000 new chemicals per year), we would never get abreast of the problem.

The fact is that there is one absolute constraint on the length of time that a scientist can devote to researching a particular problem – and that is when the grant runs out.

It is in the nature of science that always 'more research is needed'. Uncertainties, as we have seen earlier, always exist. It is for research scientists to dig out facts and throw up hypotheses, and it is for society to become familiar with the facts, evaluate them and decide what to do about them. It is not acceptable for society to live in dangerous conditions while politicians wait for scientists to arrive at consensus. If there is reasonable cause to suspect a problem with an environmental agent, the onus should be on the polluter to bring forward evidence of innocence, rather than on the victims to do the 'impossible' and 'prove' guilt. In legal terms, the burden of proof should shift from the criminal criterion of 'innocent until proved beyond reasonable doubt to be guilty' to the civil criterion of 'balance of probabilities'. In the meantime, action must be taken to protect people from the suspect agent. This is the precautionary principle, and is especially consistent with criterion number 8 in the list on p. 147.

The scientific method is an invaluable tool in the investigation of illness in society. Science is a useless object of worship, a bad master, but a good servant.

Surprisingly, in practice, the method chosen by government-appointed scientists to investigate pollution is not scientific but scholastic. Science proceeds by observation, hypothesis formation and attempts to destroy the hypothesis by experimentation. The scholastic method proceeds by comparing new facts with accepted 'knowledge', discarding the facts if they do not accord with the books.

Two cardinal cases illustrate this point – Seascale and Camelford. In the case of Seascale, a working party under the chairmanship of Sir Douglas Black was set up in 1983 to look into the alleged cluster of cancer cases in Seascale, near the Sellafield nuclear reprocessing and nuclear weapons materials factory. He found that there was an 'unusual but not unique' incidence of leukaemia in young people in the village. The report did not say so, but the chance of these cases being produced by coincidence would be about one in a million.

This observation would suggest the hypothesis that 'the leukaemias are caused by physical agents in the vicinity'. The second observation in the case is that the children of Seascale were exposed to a high level of radionuclides in the environment. Radionuclide elements are rare in nature. They are taken into the body and there emit radiation often of the, more damaging, alpha kind. This fact suggests the hypothesis that 'the leukaemias are caused by the radionuclides'. According to the scientific method, further research should have been put in hand to attempt to disprove this hypothesis.

However, in the report itself the causation hypothesis was rejected on the grounds that the expected rates of leukaemia, which are theoretical calculations based on assumptions of release rates, estimates of received doses and assumptions about the relative biological effectiveness (leukaemia-causing potential) of alpha radiation, are only one-fortieth of the dose thought to be needed to produce the observed damage. In other words, the reasoning was that there were more leukaemias than theory would predict, the theory was right, and therefore the radiation was not the cause. The corollary to this reasoning is that the higher the leukaemia incidence at Seascale, the more innocent the radiation. This is perverse, since radiation is known to be able to cause leukaemia in humans. The perversity arises because the method used was not scientific but scholastic. It assumed that all we need to know about radiation is in the textbooks, and that new findings are to be compared with the textbooks, rather than the textbooks to be compared with new observations. The unscientific nature of the logic is clinched by the nuclear scientists' argument that more cases would be required to make a statistically significant cluster. More cases would on this logic mean that Sellafield was more innocent. This would mean that the hypothesis that 'the Sellafield emissions did not cause the leukaemias' was unfalsifiable, and therefore not scientific.

This line of official reasoning was repeated in the case of the Camelford disaster, known officially as the Lowermoor incident. On 6 July 1988, 20 tonnes of concentrated aluminium sulphate solution were discharged into the treated water reservoir at Lowermoor, Cornwall, which serves the town of Camelford. Local residents and holidaymakers who drank the water experienced a variety of acute effects, and a lesser number also remained ill for a long time thereafter. Six months later a committee was set up under Dame Barbara Clayton to provide independent expert advice to the Secretary of State for Health.[3] The group noted that this incident was unique in the history of pollution; there was no previous experience of humans taking in this particular cocktail of ionic lead, zinc, copper, aluminium and sulphate. They also noted that the symptoms of the people were also unique. They had wide-ranging problems: sore/dry mouth, fatigue, malaise, stomach aches, extreme thirst, nausea and vomiting, itching, sore eyes and mouth ulcers. The persistent effects noted by the group were aches and joint pains, memory loss, poor concentration, speech problems, depression and behavioural problems in children, hypersensitivity, rashes and mouth ulcers and gastrointestinal disorders. These symptoms do not fit into any recognized diagnostic category. So the observation is a unique toxic assault, and a unique resultant syndrome.

It was hypothesized that the toxins caused the illness. Surprisingly, instead of testing this hypothesis by advising on necessary medical and scientific studies, the group opened their textbooks, and looked up the effects of each of the ions as they are known in isolation. In each case they found that the ion in those concentrations was incapable of causing those effects. On this evidence (book-based scholastic theory that did not relate to mixtures of ions) they concluded that the cocktail was incapable of causing the illness. There was scientific evidence of deposition of aluminium in the bones of one affected patient. The group specifically advised against following up this lead. The group concluded that its book learning could not account for the illness and that, ergo, the symptoms were due to 'anxiety'. There was no psychiatrist in the group to advise on this point. As a result of the public outcry that followed, the Clayton Group was reconvened, and came to the conclusion that they had been quite right in the first place.

Years later, the affected citizens were given out-of-court settlements in compensation for their suffering. This incident occurred when South West Water was being prepared for privatization.

It emerges from this that the statements of scientists, especially those working at the behest of government, are not necessarily 'scientific' but instead statements based on 'authority'. The charitable view is that the confusion comes about not through cynicism or bad faith, but because in the complexity of detail the simplicities of the method are lost to view.

# IMMUNE SYSTEM

The immune system provides the body's defensive interface with the environment. It is an exceedingly complex web of chemicals, cells and communications which lies at the boundary of our selves and our physical and chemical environment. It has the task of surveying all the substances in our skin, respiratory system, digestive tract, tissues and blood 24 hours a day, 365 days a year, and deciding what is, and what is not, a threat to our well-being. It must pick up infecting and infesting agents and kill them, but should not attack neutral substances such as bits of dust and food. It must identify and kill body cells that have mutated to a cancerous form, but must not attack healthy cells and tissues which constitute the body. For the most part it gets this job done without fuss requiring only that its defences be not overwhelmed, that it is part of a reasonably happy person and that it is treated to adequate fresh foods and given a judicious balance between rest and activity. Sometimes if it is presented with a strong challenge, such as an influenza virus, it requires us to switch off the brain, cease to exert physically and take to our beds for a few days so that blood can be diverted exclusively to the immune system while it solves the problem. Not a lot to ask, but often this is denied it.

The immune system is second only to the brain in complexity. Some cells in the immune system, for example some T-lymphocytes, are derived from the same embryonic tissues that gave rise to the brain and the rest of the central nervous system and these chemicals serve as intermediaries between brain and body defence. A new science has sprung up, psycho–neuro–immunology, to study the complex interrelationships between the mind and the immune defences of the body that it inhabits. The special T-lymphocytes respond to the same chemical neurotransmitters that stimulate nerve cells, and may be seen as the interface between our consciousness and our immune system.

## How the immune system works

The workings of the system have been set out with clarity in *Hayfever: The Complete Guide* by Dr Jonathan Brostoff and Linda Gamlin.[4]

This is how it works in highly simplified steps (Figure 8.1).

1 Infants are born with hundreds of thousands of antibodies; Y-shaped protein molecules which can bind themselves to foreign proteins (called antigens).
2 Certain immune cells called T-suppressor lymphocytes control these antibodies in the infant, preventing them from attacking and damaging items which do not constitute a threat. Some chemicals, for instance nitrogen dioxide, can impair this process.

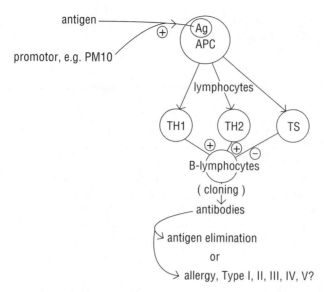

**Figure 8.1** The immune system (simplified).

3 In the adult, foreign protein (antigen) is seized by antigen-presenting cells, chewed up and presented to T-lymphocytes for consideration. As well as T-suppressors, T-helper cells examine the material. (These are the cells which are knocked out by AIDS.) If they decide that the antigen is a threat, they will instruct another class of cell, the B-lymphocyte, to produce antibodies to the antigen.

4 There are two kinds of T-helper cells: TH1 and TH2. TH1 cells cause B-lymphocytes to produce antibodies which react gently but effectively with the antigen. TH2 cells cause the production of IgE antibodies by the B-lymphocytes, which causes a violent reaction. Mast cells will release histamine and several other chemicals that cause inflammation (swelling and congestion) of the tissues and contraction of nearby smooth muscles. It is thought that the purpose of this reaction is to expel parasites such as worms from the intestines. Unfortunately, for many sufferers, it is the reaction at the root of allergic reactions such as hayfever, asthma, eczema and possibly irritable bowel syndrome (IBS).

Four distinct types of allergic reaction are recognized by immunologists. Type V is suggested here as a hypothetical cause of the kind of disorder which is treated by clinical ecologists (physicians who study intolerance to food and chemicals).

Given the complexity of the system and the tasks it is asked to perform, it is surprising that the immune system does not go wrong more often. Sometimes it is simply overwhelmed by the attack of an infecting agent, with the result that the individual dies. Less drastic failures are set out in Table 8.1 and detailed in the next section.

# Allergic disease

Allergy is well known as hayfever, and its close relative perennial rhinitis, which occurs at any time of year. Allergy also is one of the co-factors that results in asthma, and is involved in some forms of eczema or dermatitis. In allergy, the immune system has, as it were, got hold of the wrong idea. In its continuous search for threats to the system, it has picked up a piece of pollen, house dust, house dust mite faeces, or other substance, and has decided that it must be fought. It is a kind of biological paranoia. However, the mistake is understandable, because the goalposts in the allergy game are being widened and moved all the time.

## Hayfever and asthma

Allergic disease has been on the increase since the early 1800s. Allergy to horses was known in ancient Greece, but hayfever was not described until 1819. It began in aristocrats and in urban populations, and spread slowly down the social ladder. This pattern is reflected in the present day, allergy being consistently more frequent in urban societies than in rural and traditional populations. It affects the only child and the firstborn child four times more often than it affects other children. It is thought that the increased rate of colds experienced by children with siblings has a protective effect against allergy.

Animals get allergies, but they do not get hayfever. The reason for this is not known. Air pollution is a candidate, explaining the urban siting and the recent spread to rural areas as cars take pollution further afield – although this does not necessarily explain the increases in allergy seen in remote islands. Soot particles

**Table 8.1**  Disorders of immune function

| | |
|---|---|
| 1 | Allergy |
| | Hayfever/rhinitis |
| | Asthma |
| | Eczema |
| | ?Irritable bowel syndrome |
| 2 | Multiple sensitivity, chemical and food intolerance |
| 3 | Autoimmune conditions |
| 4 | Post-viral fatigue syndrome |
| 5 | Immune disorder syndrome |
| 6 | Acquired immunodeficiency syndrome (AIDS) |

are known to enhance the production of IgE. But pollution does not explain the vulnerability of aristocrats and only/eldest children. Brostoff and Gamlin[4] define the required culprit thus:

> ... it is tempting to look for some aspect of modern living that was first enjoyed only by the very wealthy, but then gradually spread to the middle classes, and is now available to all sectors of our egalitarian society. If that luxury item was something which could irritate the nose, or subtly influence the immune system of a young child, it might qualify as a suspect.

Interestingly, perfumes fit this bill fairly well. Aristocrats would have used more perfume, and the environment of eldest and only children is considerably more fragrant than a house full of children, where the mother tends to give up on trying to keep the place in tip-top cleanliness. The strong, synthetic 'fresh' perfumes are designed to stimulate the nose strongly, and many people feel they actually irritate the nose. This can only be an hypothesis at this stage.

As well as hayfever, asthma is also on the increase. It is often argued that air pollution has been falling since the great smogs of the 1950s whereas asthma is rising, and that therefore the two cannot be linked. This does not necessarily follow, since the type of air pollution has changed. Instead of the dense smogs caused by burning coal, we breathe the new haze caused by road traffic, with a new profile of pollutants. Whatever the cause of the increase in asthma cases, there is little doubt that traffic pollution makes established asthmatics wheeze more. We will return to this topic in chapter 11.

# Multiple sensitivity, chemical and food intolerance

## Co-development

The human immune system has developed over the course of some 2 million years, on the top of a mammalian immune system that goes back some 40 million years. In that time the system has faced a number of changes and challenges, and has co-developed with, and therefore adapted to, the prevailing injurious agents, whether irritative, infective, infestational or allergenic. It has even co-developed with naturally occurring forms of radiation. In that time it has had to adapt to two forms of chemicals: simple chemicals such as salts and other ions and organic chemicals which have been produced by living systems. Some of the latter are highly toxic, often designedly so; for instance, ricin produced by the castor oil bean is one of the most powerful poisons known. But all of these substances, whether beneficial, neutral, injurious or highly toxic, share two characteristics: we have co-developed with them and they are the products of living systems. Over the last century, this situation has changed.

# The chemical challenge

Towards the end of the first 2 million years of human evolution, we began to get clever with chemicals. The Greeks, Arabs and mediaeval alchemists dabbled in chemistry, but serious chemical production began in the nineteenth century, so that by about 1890 there were about 150 chemicals available with which the average urbanized human could be expected to come into contact. Four generations later that number has multiplied by a factor of 460, so that we now have some 70 000 chemicals in our environment, with another 1000–2000 being added each year, many of them in everyday, intimate contact. This represents a huge shift in our ecological niche in a very short time and a severe challenge to our immune system. This is not mere speculation: some 200 occupational agents are recognized by occupational physicians as being capable of causing asthma.[5]

It is in part true that there is no intrinsic difference between a natural and a synthetic molecule. Ascorbic acid (vitamin C) from an orange has exactly the same effect in the body as ascorbic acid produced in a vat in the Roche Laboratories. Natural vitamin C from an orange may be assisted in its absorption by the presence of co-produced substances, but the principle remains that synthetic compounds do not necessarily differ in themselves from natural compounds of the same structure. They are all chemicals.

Where they do differ is that, whereas natural compounds have originated from enzymes produced by living systems, and are therefore capable of being broken down by enzymes produced by living systems, synthetic compounds may not necessarily be susceptible to this kind of biodegredation. DDT is the best-known example of this characteristic. Every school child now knows that this persistent pesticide can be detected in the fat of Antarctic penguins, and that unless a bacterium eventually develops the ability to break down DDT it will still be detectable hundreds of years from now.

This longevity of non-biodegradable substances is part of the problem with the notorious 'ozone-eating' CFCs which are composed of chlorine, with its more reactive cousin fluorine, locked on to a couple of carbon atoms. The chlorine–carbon bond is chemists' stock-in-trade. If a drug is promising, but fails to stay long enough in the body, a chlorine atom is attached to a carbon atom on this or that corner, with the result that the body cannot clear it so quickly. To a chemist, this is fundamental practice. In nature, only two chemicals contain the chlorine–carbon bond, and one of them is ricin, the poison in the castor oil bean. This does not mean that all synthetic carbon–chlorine compounds are toxic, merely that they are unusual and unfamiliar to our defence systems. In principle, they may pose a problem for our immune system. Although they are man-made, synthetic chemicals are not human, and do not qualify for human rights. They are not 'innocent until proved guilty'. They should be treated in a precautionary way, that is the onus of proof should be on the manufacturers to show that they do not harm life, rather than on the victims of the illness they produce to 'prove' that they have been harmed by them.

# The effects on humans

Clinical ecologists, doctors who are represented by the British Society for Allergy and Environmental Medicine,[a] have for a long time been treating people who react adversely to a variety of artificial chemicals. This form of medicine suffered a brief spell of notoriety in the media when the tabloids picked up a case of a young singer who they dubbed as 'allergic to the twentieth century'. The furore about this case did nothing to help the credibility of the young discipline of clinical ecology with medicine as a whole, and the tabloid journalists, as is their wont, soon became bored with the topic, having done it to death in the eyes of the public and certainly in the eyes of the medical profession. Meanwhile, scientific research continues into the reaction of individuals to new chemicals, but is limited by the difficulty of obtaining funds for research. The big money in medical research is in drugs. Clinical ecology offers cures not by taking drugs but by avoiding chemicals and foods that cause problems. Therefore there is a difficulty in getting funded.

Terminology also caused a problem. In the 1970s, the term 'food allergy' was used to describe the problem that some patients had with foods. Immunologists objected that there were four recognized types of allergy, none of which fitted the pattern that ecologists were treating. This problem was neatly overcome by switching to 'food intolerance' as a descriptive term.

Surveys of food intolerance in populations show wide variations in proportions varying from 1% to 30% affected. The work of Dr Joseph Egger at Great Ormond Street Hospitals (see p. 198) has done much to establish the credibility of intolerance to food additives as a cause of childhood hyperactivity in the scientific community. Meanwhile, the sheer pragmatism of parents and general practitioners, as more and more learn that many hyperactive children respond well to a diet rigorously free of coal tar dyes, is affecting what food manufacturers are prepared to put in their foods.

# Autoimmune conditions

Sometimes the body's defences turn against themselves. Rheumatoid arthritis is the commonest of these conditions, and results from a side-effect of natural antibodies designed to kill a certain streptococcus. The antibodies also attack the collagen in joints. It is a disease of modern times, since 1800, but is becoming less common now, possibly because better social conditions have lessened the prevalence of streptococcal infections, possibly because the streptococcus has mutated, or possibly because penicillin means that infections are shorter and less severe.

[a] BSAEM, with the British Society for Nutritional Medicine, PO Box 28, Totton, Southampton SO4 22A, UK.

Scleroderma is an autoimmune disorder in which new chemicals are clearly implicated. Silicone breast implants, vinyl chloride, dapsone (an anti-leprosy drug) and paraffin can all induce the immune system to turn on the body, with the result of inflammation of muscles, and frequent 'dead fingers'.

# Post-viral fatigue syndrome

Post-viral fatigue syndrome (PVFS), also known as myalgic encephalomyelitis (ME), has been recognized since the beginning of the twentieth century under a variety of names (Royal Free disease, neurasthenia). Controversy still surrounds the criteria which must be met to warrant the diagnosis. Whatever the exact status of the disease, there is no doubt that the numbers of people affected have exploded in the last decade. It is estimated that there are 150 000 affected individuals in the UK, of whom 24 000 are school children. These estimates are liable to inaccuracy, since ME is not recognized, let alone officially reported, by many doctors. The condition is characterized by exercise-induced fatigue, depression of brain function and a course that fluctuates from hour to hour and day to day. The diagnosis is made by the presence of fatigue after exercise, with muscle weakness, pain, tenderness and twitching (fasciculation), impaired concentration and short-term memory, sleep impairment and emotional lability (ups and downs occurring at short notice). A variety of other symptoms occurs, including sweating, abnormal heart rhythm, nausea, stomach disturbances and problems with passing water. It often follows a challenge to the immune system such as infection (viral infections are thought to have triggered 75% of cases), vaccination (which is thought to trigger about 3% of cases) or emotionally traumatic events. It is thought that the syndrome results from the body failing to complete the process of response to an infection, so that high levels of defence chemicals called cytokines are still in circulation and produce the symptoms.

Most but not all doctors now recognize this as a true syndrome rather than something that is all in the mind. The difficulty is that there is no 'gold standard' diagnostic test to clinch the diagnosis. It is likely that a number of different subsets of the disease will be laid out eventually, and it is possible that some but not all of the cases will be found to have been psychological in origin. If PVFS were a somatization reaction ('all in the mind'), subtle changes in illness behaviour would be detectable. Fifteen per cent of patients with chronic fatigue do show this behaviour, but a study in Leeds found no difference in illness behaviour between chronic fatigue patients and multiple sclerosis patients.[6] Post-viral fatigue syndrome does therefore offer inconclusive but worrying evidence that the competence of our immune systems may be beginning to fail.

# Acquired immunodeficiency syndrome (AIDS)

Acquired immunodeficiency syndrome is well known as the viral infection which spread from monkeys to humans in the 1950s and is now spreading among humans through sexual contact and shared needles. Nobody yet knows why it suddenly jumped the species barrier. Theories have included a mutation caused by the heavy radioactive fallout into the tropical rainforests from atom bomb tests in the 1950s and deliberate germ warfare experiments (the CIA is on record as expressing in the 1950s that there was a need for an agent that attacks the immune system) but there is not sufficient evidence to gain general acceptability for either of these theories. Much has been made of some interesting exceptions to the accepted theory that the disease is caused by the HIV retrovirus – for instance, not every AIDS patient shows evidence of HIV infection. These exceptions are by no means sufficient to undermine the rule that sexual behaviour must change towards fidelity and safe sex in order to curb the spread of the infection.

Right-wing commentators have challenged the amount spent on AIDS, suggesting that it is excessive. The expenditure is justified when we remember that if the disease continues to spread, especially through heterosexual activity, the proportion of the population affected will grow exponentially, that is the rate of increase will grow from year to year.

# DETOXIFICATION

Detoxification is the name given to the process by which the body deals with unwanted chemicals, whether natural or artificial. In phase 1 detoxification, enzymes, mainly in the liver, alter the unwanted molecule by oxidation, reduction, hydrolysis or hydration. Phase 2 detoxification adds a 'polar group' to the substance, often after preliminary alterations by phase 1 processes. The polar group usually means that the resultant combination is more water-soluble. Phase 2 consists of sulphation, glucuronidation, glutathione conjugation, acetylation, amino acid conjugation or methylation.

It is possible that detoxification systems may become overloaded by the increased burden of chemicals in our environment, especially if combined with nutritional deficiencies.

Glutathione conjugation is a clearance pathway that seems to be most likely to become a bottleneck. The enzymes that run the show, glutathione peroxidase and glutathione transferase, are unique in requiring a trace element, selenium, both in their structure and as a co-factor in their function, and they also require two uncommon sulphur-bearing amino acids. There is therefore a risk that these enzymes will be unable to operate maximally in people who are not optimally nourished. These enzymes are important: they are involved in the antioxidant pathways that clear up free radicals (see below) and also in clearing pesticides and drugs from the body. The response of these enzymes to overload and therapy with glutathione and selenium can be measured.[b]

[b] Dr John McLaren Howard, Biolab Medical Unit, Weymouth Street, London, personal communication.

## SYNERGY OR THE COCKTAIL EFFECT

The main tool of science in approaching a complex field is to attempt to isolate one variable in order to determine its effect. Faced with the problem of finding how a motor works, a scientist might remove a spark plug and discover that the engine can still run, but less smoothly. Removing the high-tension lead, he will find that it is vital to the function, and so on. This is a valid method, but is excruciatingly slow when applied to complex systems, and sometimes, as we have seen in the case of the Camelford scandal, it leads to unjustified results.

Biological systems are far more complex than motors. They flow like rivers cascading over rocks, but with each movement the nature of the river changes. One rock may produce one alteration of flow, but, depending on its site, the position and nature of another rock may magnify or possibly neutralize the alteration.

For instance, both smoking and asbestos are known to cause lung cancer. But if a man both smokes and inhales asbestos, his risk is not doubled, it is increased by a factor of 20. The two factors work together: there is synergy. The same holds true for smoking and radon gas exposure, in which case the risk of lung cancer increases by a factor of ten.

We are bathed in a cocktail of chemicals, many of which are known to have adverse effects at high doses. We try to control these effects by setting standards, limiting the dose expected to mere fractions of the levels at which we know that effects appear. Say that the level for 100 agents is set at one-hundredth of that which is harmful, and a person is exposed to the whole lot. If their effects merely add up arithmetically one to the other, the person is already at risk: but if even two or three act synergistically, like tobacco and asbestos, the safety level is breached. Figure 8.2 shows the possible synergic effects of a sample of common pollutants.

This list is by no means exhaustive, but shows the potential for unexpected effects and interaction to take place. There is scope for far more research into this problem, and there is certainly no room for complacency about the safety of the standard levels that are set.

## FREE RADICALS

Anyone in possession of a GCSE in chemistry will remember that chlorine and hydrogen peroxide owe their bleaching properties to their ability to split oxygen, $O_2$, into two atoms of charged atomic oxygen, $O^-$, which is highly reactive, combining with the nearest available substance. In the body, this activated oxygen and other molecules with similar properties are referred to as 'free radicals'. They have a role in the normal defence process, being created by white cells in the process of inflammation that accompanies infection. Adrenaline and noradrenaline, released during periods of stress, increase their production.

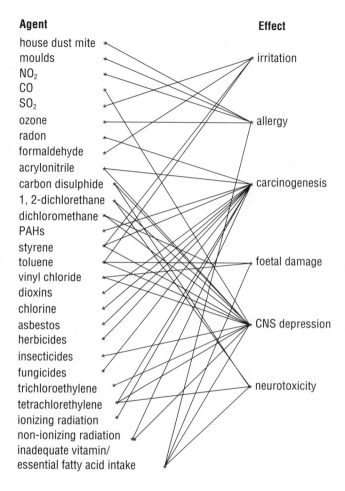

**Figure 8.2** Synergy.

Some pollutants are known to increase the levels of free radicals:

- cigarette smoke
- photochemical smog from traffic
- fine particles
- ozone
- nitrogen dioxide
- peroxyacyl nitrites
- excess iron and copper
- radiation.

The effects of free radical release in the body are:

- inflammation
- ageing
- atherogenesis (deposition of cholesterol in the arteries)
- degenerative arthritis
- alterations in immune reactions
- cancer
- diminished intracellular magnesium
- nerve degeneration, e.g. Parkinson's disease.

In order to mop-up free radicals, the body needs the 'antioxidant' vitamins A, C and E, plus selenium, copper, manganese and zinc. As will be shown in chapter 10, levels of many of these substances are relatively deficient in a highly processed diet. An enzyme derived from cows, bovine sulphoxide dismutase, is being used experimentally to scavenge free radicals.

# STRESS

Stress in physics describes the changes in a structure that come about in response to an external load. The term has been imported into human psychology to describe our responses to the many loads that life places on us. Small amounts of stress help us to work at optimal efficiency, but excessive stress causes inefficient functioning and makes us prone to illness. There is a large amount of overlap between the concept of stress and the psychiatric description of anxiety, which is an emotional response to perceived threat. The difference lies in the fact that stress deals with external loads, whereas anxiety includes a response to emotions arising from activity within the person's consciousness, which may be relatively independent of external conditions.

Selye has described the following types of strategy commonly used in response to stress:[7]

- accepting
- tolerating
- avoiding
- minimizing.

If these strategies are not sufficient, the individual will need support in order to cope with the stress.

## Stress and the immune system

The physiological purpose of stress or anxiety, as every schoolchild knows, is to prepare us for 'fight or flight'. Adrenaline and noradrenaline are released by the adrenal medulla as a short-term response, and the steroid cortisol released from the adrenal cortex controls longer term reactions. In nature, the energy generated by adrenaline is dissipated in physical activity. Modern life, although stressful, does not offer much scope for physical activity. It is thought that the effects of the stress hormones are therefore expressed in increased muscle tension, increased blood pressure and emotional irritability. There is also an effect on the immune system. There is an intimate connection between the nervous system and the immune system. The autonomic nervous system, which controls the internal organs, including heart and blood vessels, also innervates the spleen and bone marrow, tissues that are home to the immune system. Some of the T-lymphocytes are derived from the 'neural crest', the same embryonic tissues that give rise to the brain and nervous system. These T-lymphocyte cells have neurotransmitter receptors just like nerve cells, and produce peptides called cytokines (production of which can be influenced by cortisol from the adrenal gland). These cells can be seen as the conscious controllers of our body's defences, the interface between mind and body. It is now understandable how periods of mental stress can result in physical illness.

Evidence to back this mechanism comes from the observation that the incidence of herpes simplex (cold sores) increased among students who were stressed by examination.[8] It is known that cortisol can suppress some defence reactions. Normally cortisol production is automatically limited by a negative feedback mechanism: when levels are high, further production is switched off. Dexamethasone is a steroid drug that mimics this negative feedback on cortisol production. Some people with depression do not show this negative feedback in response to dexamethasone – they are called non-suppressors. Stress induced a temporary non-suppressor status in the students, which lowers the activity of the 'natural killer' lymphocytes and lymphocyte proliferation, which resulted in the herpes virus outbreaks.

The behaviour of the immune system can be conditioned in a classical Pavlovian way. In one experiment, mice were given cyclophosphamide together with saccharin several times.[9] Cyclophosphamide suppresses the immune system. When they were then given saccharin alone, the immune system again showed signs of suppression – a classic conditioned response.

## Stress in modern life

Every aspect of existence can generate stress in us.[c]

- Preoccupation with time causes stress not only through our obsession with fulfilling the requirements of an overfull diary, but also because we are all conscious that time will in the end lead us to death. Many of our psychological defence mechanisms are devoted to denial of this 'mortal fear'. We have inverted Victorian values. They were morbidly fascinated with death, but banished sex from their conscious lives: we are morbidly fascinated with sex, but

[c] The classification used here is derived from the philosopher Herman Dooyeweerd.

try to deny the reality of death. We attempt to control death by technologizing terminal illness, and paradoxically seek to found our national security on nuclear deterrence, which is nothing but the threat of death on a global scale.

- Space or lack of it creates stress through overcrowding. Large cities are attractive to the young because they are stimulating. It has been found that the speed at which people walk on the pavement is proportional to the size of the city. Overstimulation leads to exhaustion.
- Energy in any of its forms is stressful in excess: cold, heat and noise. Kinetic energy, especially in the form of the motor car and other fast-moving machines, causes trauma and death.
- Matter in the form of stimulant chemicals – drugs, including caffeine and alcohol, increase stress when taken in excess or by people who are sensitive to their effects.
- Life demands that certain basic needs are fulfilled – water, food, shelter, warmth and hygiene. Other life forms from sabre-toothed tigers to human beings with whom we do not see eye to eye may threaten our sense of security.
- Psychological states are the final common pathway for all other stressants. Relationships in the past – early family dynamics and traumas – affect present situations, often in a dysfunctional way.
- Social relationships – exclusion, oppression, dependency – have very powerful effects.
- Economic situations are a prime cause of stress, primarily to the poor, but also to wealthy people when they feel that wealth is threatened.
- Aesthetic or rather dysaesthetic conditions – noise, ugliness, conflict – cause stress.
- Juridical stresses arise both from the sense of guilt, whether realistic or psychological, and also from the operation of law on the individual, especially if justice is miscarried.
- Ethical: the need to feel loved is fundamental to our existence. Unconditional love often appears to be in short supply.
- Central: a sense of purpose gives life its ultimate security. Many people are caught in a pincer movement between philosophical vacuity at one extreme and worklessness at the other. Many live in an atmosphere of pointlessness and seek to find happiness in immediate gratification of the senses, or to express their anger in violence. Some escape from the frying pan of this anomie into the fire of one or another of the many fundamentalisms on offer, there to suffer the stresses of exclusivity, regimentation and, only too often, conflict.

All of this suffering seems a pity when life itself, in whatever aspect it is seen, offers a challenging and satisfying purpose in learning how to live happily in such a way that others, including our descendants, are also able to live happily.

# REFERENCES

1    Carson R (1963) *Silent Spring.* Hamish Hamilton, London.

2    Bradford Hill A (1965) *The Environment and Disease: Association or Causation?* Proceedings of Royal Society of Medicine. January 14.

3    The Lowermoor Incident Advisory Group (1989) *Water Pollution at Lowermoor, North Cornwall.* Cornwall and Isles of Scilly Health Authority, London.

4    Brostoff J and Gamlin L (1993) *Hayfever: The Complete Guide.* Bloomsbury, London.

5    Bardana E J (1995) Occupational asthma and related respiratory disorders. *Disease-a-Month:* **41(3)**; 143–99.

6    Trigwell P, Hatcher S, Johnson M *et al.* (1995) Abnormal illness behaviour in chronic fatigue syndrome and multiple sclerosis. *BMJ:* **311**; 15–18.

7    Selye H (1975) Confusion and controversy in the stress field. *J Human Stress:* **1(2)**; 37–44.

8    Glaser R, Kiecolt-Glaser J K, Speicher C E *et al.* (1985) Stress, loneliness and changes in Herpes virus latency. *J Behav Med:* **8(3)**; 249–60.

9    Neven P J, Dantzer R, Le Moal M (1986) Behaviourally conditioned suppression of nitrogen-induced lymphoproliferation and antibody production in mice. *Neuro Lett:* **65(3)**; 293–8.

# 9

# Pollution by air, water and land

*The most important effects of pollution are extremely delayed and indirect.*

Rene Dubos[1]

## AIR POLLUTION

On a day-to-day basis the weight of air we breathe is ten times heavier than the weight of water that we drink. Carried in this air are a wide variety of bacteria, viruses, fungal spores, miscellaneous bits of debris, smoke particles and vapours, any or all of which may affect our health. This fact may be seized on triumphantly by health advice cynics who predict that it is only a matter of time before experts are advising that breathing is bad for you.

## TOBACCO SMOKING

It took 20 years of intensive research and some 50 000 scientific papers for the scientific community to agree that smoking is without doubt one of the foremost health problems of our time. Even now, diehards in the tobacco industry are contending that the matter is 'not conclusively proved' and that smoking has beneficial effects through the relaxation that it induces, and that until recently it had no convincing evidence that nicotine is a drug of addiction. The mainstream view, however, is that tobacco smoking is not only the most serious form of air pollution, but also the greatest single health threat of modern times.

### Tobacco advertising

Smoking costs the NHS £437 million per year in efforts spent trying to remedy the damage wrought by smoking. It is estimated that 100 000 people in the UK die per year as a result of smoking-related diseases. For these reasons, the medical, nursing and caring professions – in fact anyone with an interest in health, and including many honest nicotine addicts – are united in wishing to see every discouragement brought to bear on smoking. During the consultation period for the Health of the Nation process, the request was made repeatedly that the advertisement of tobacco products should be banned. So great was the pressure that the Department of Health commissioned a report from its own economics and operational research division on the effect of tobacco advertising on tobacco consumption.[2] Their conclusion:

> The balance of evidence [from year to year variations in advertising expenditure within countries] thus supports the conclusion that advertising does have a positive effect on consumption.

Regarding the effects of advertising bans in other countries, they concluded:

> ... the current evidence available on these four countries (Norway, Finland, Canada and New Zealand) indicates a significant effect. In each case the banning of advertising was followed by a fall in smoking on a scale which cannot reasonably be attributed to other factors.

The fall in tobacco consumption achieved in New Zealand was thought to be about 5.5%, in Canada about 4%, in Finland 6.7% and Norway 9%. The greatest effect is expected to be seen in the next generation, since there is evidence that tobacco advertising has a particular influence on children. The Department of Health report noted that 'there is a great deal of evidence to show that young people recognise tobacco advertisements and that those who go on to smoke are more likely to recognise them'.

The evidence that advertising does increase consumption comes from New Zealand, where before the ban was introduced the tobacco industry increased its advertising budget by 14%. Shortly after this, tobacco consumption increased by 4.3% and the number of smokers by 2.6%.[3] This fact overturns the contention of the tobacco industry that advertising merely persuades people to shift from one brand to another. If this were really the case, it would clearly be in the best immediate financial interest of the industry to call a ceasefire in the advertising war, since it is spending an estimated £100 million per year on it.

In the end, it is plain that, if the tobacco industry is to continue to exist or to grow, it needs to replace the smokers who die at a rate of 100 000 per year as a result of their addiction. For this reason, it is unfortunately necessary for them to recruit young people, and advertising is one of the means that enables this to happen – the other being the powerfully addictive effect of nicotine itself.

Another side-effect of the Conservative Government's failure to ban tobacco advertising is to undermine the commitment of the medical profession to health promotion. Consciously or unconsciously, the GP will reason, 'since the government is not serious about smoking cessation, why should I put effort into it?'

# Why no ban?

Since it is the case that tobacco damages health, and smoking reduction, as well as several smoking-related diseases, are Health of the Nation key areas, and since the government's own advisers are giving it such a clear message, the question arises, 'why does the government not ban tobacco advertising?'.

In answer to this question cynics often mention the fact that the tax revenue to the Treasury from tobacco products is about £5 billion per year, and also that by killing off pensioners, the state is saved billions in pension payouts. (The flow of money is not all one way; since 1980, £33 million of taxpayers' money has gone to support the tobacco industry in Northern Ireland, and the EU gives large subsidies to its tobacco growers.) The inference is that government does not in fact wish to curtail tobacco use as it is just as addicted to the tobacco tax revenues as the smoker is to tobacco itself. This argument might have some weight if it could be expected that tobacco sales would collapse overnight as the result of a ban, but, as we have seen, the effects are far more gradual than that. Since nicotine is so addictive, the Treasury can be certain of a significant minority of addicts that it can sponge off for years to come. Any reductions in tobacco revenue as a result of an advertising ban or other health measures can easily be made up through taxation on other polluting processes.

In 1971, an inquiry set up with Treasury, Customs and Excise, Department of Trade and Industry and Department of Health and Social Security officials found that a 20% reduction in smoking over a 30-year period would result in a saving of 250 000 lives, but that this saving would cost an extra £12 million in social security payments. This is a trifling sum in the scale of government spending (equivalent to four days' spending on the futile Trident nuclear fleet) and is certainly not sufficient to deter the government from trying to reduce smoking.

A more recent report[4] showed that a 40% reduction in cigarette consumption would create up to 150 000 jobs because of the 'responding' effect of the money saved on cigarettes, which would go on cars, petrol, recreation, entertainment, education and consumer goods. This would more than compensate for the 4000 jobs lost out of the 12 000 workers directly employed by the cigarette industry. Since the relation between smoking reduction and jobs created is linear, a 5% cut from a ban on advertising could create 18 750 jobs.

Why, then, does government not ban tobacco advertising? In February 1994 it was reported that Paul Flynn MP had in his possession a letter from Peter Middleton, sales and marketing director of Imperial Tobacco, to the Prime Minister, John Major. The letter states that the Conservative Party had been given the opportunity to use 2000 advertising sites in the 1992 election 'because they were the only party that stated in their manifesto that they would vote against the proposed EU directive on the banning of tobacco advertising'. The Prime Minister made no relevant reply when Mr Flynn asked him whether he would promise never again to take money, bribes or favours from the tobacco industry. In the letter, Middleton states that the Conservative Party paid for the sites. It is not known how much they paid, but by paying something it was possible for the position to be defended, as for example by Tim Smith MP, then vice-chairman of the Conservative Party, when he wrote to me on 30 October 1992, 'It is not true that the Conservative Party was *given* advertising space by the tobacco industry in the last election' [emphasis added].

Of course, the pressure on government comes not only from the tobacco industry, but also from the advertising industry, which benefits greatly from advertising tobacco products.

The conclusion is that when political parties are beholden to large corporations, public policy (in this case an effective fight against the addictive drug nicotine) is hamstrung.

---

### Recommendation

1   The financial accounts of political parties must be made fully available for public inspection.
2   Serious consideration must be given to the possibility of political parties being funded from the public purse at rates proportional to their membership, and for any donation to be made to them from corporate bodies to be strictly regulated to avoid undue influence.

---

# INDOOR AIR QUALITY

Most of us spend more than 90% of our lives indoors, bathed in a sea of pollutants concentrated by the entrapped air, and exacerbated by the chemicals we add to kill the odours that we create. Chief among the polluters is the house dust mite.

## House dust mite

House dust mites are microscopic creatures that feed on flakes of human skin that we shed naturally. Their faeces are highly allergenic to humans, and the allergy can manifest as asthma, rhinitis (constant blocked nose and sneezing) and eczema, all of which conditions have been increasing in recent years. Eczema is the crown of the mite's repertoire, since it causes more skin cell shedding, and therefore obtains for itself more food.

There has been a 5% increase in the population of house dust mites between 1980 and 1990. The mites need to be humid and warm, and to have a furry environment in which to live. The recent increase in carpets, home insulation, central heating and the domestic vacuum cleaner (which is very efficient at spreading mites and their faeces) may have contributed to its population explosion. The like-lihood of having an asthmatic in the home is positively correlated with the number of house dust mites in the home. The house dust mite therefore has a strong case to answer as a co-factor in the increase in the number of cases of people with asthma.

Research is being carried out at present into the effectiveness of house dust mite avoidance measures, including acaricidal sprays that kill it, ultrafiltering vacuum cleaners and impermeable bed covers. The results should be available in 1997.

Along with house dust mite, our habit of keeping increased numbers of cats and dogs as pets may be a supporting cause of increased prevalence, since their dan-druff and hairs may also be allergenic, although the average purchase of pet food (and therefore the number of pets kept) has not increased significantly since the 1960s. House dust itself is also commonly allergenic.

## Mould spores

Mould spores are present in damp housing, thriving especially on condensation (chapter 4). It appears that we tread a narrow path between the Scylla of cold damp houses which expose us to moulds and the charybdis of overheated houses which expose us to house dust mite.

## Nitrogen dioxide

This gas is formed when domestic gas is burned. Natural North Sea gas burns at a slightly lower temperature than the old town gas, and therefore produces slightly less nitrogen dioxide. Gas cooking stoves are the main source since gas fires usually have flues to conduct the waste gases out of the room. The health effects of nitrogen dioxide at levels found in the home (as opposed to high levels used in experiments) are unclear, although at everyday levels it is associated with an increase in respiratory tract infections. Nitrogen dioxide increases the sensitivity of asthmatics to a challenging dose of house dust mite. Studies have shown that nitrogen dioxide in very high doses is capable of reducing parts of the immune system that induce tolerance.

## Carbon monoxide

Carbon monoxide is produced from gas cooking stoves in small amounts, but the main danger is from badly adjusted gas appliances and blocked flues. The gas has two main biological effects: it combines tightly with haemoglobin in the blood and it is also a neurotoxin (nerve poison). Smokers inhale carbon monoxide from tobacco, so that 3–15% of their blood is deactivated by carboxyhaemoglobin.

Levels of carbon monoxide in motor cars are four to five times higher than in ordinary outdoor air. Low-level symptoms of carbon monoxide poisoning include headaches and abdominal pain. Motor coordination becomes depressed on breathing 4% carbon monoxide, and higher levels still can lead to unconsciousness and death: this is a real risk if gas appliances are burning incompletely or if flues are blocked.

# Formaldehyde

This gas is produced in small amounts naturally, but has entered our indoor environment in a big way as a vapour given off by resins in chipboard, plywood, some insulation materials, cigarette smoke and cooking. Its concentration is about 1000 times greater indoors than in urban outdoor air.

Formaldehyde may irritate the nose at levels that can just be smelled. It may make some people, especially children, more susceptible to respiratory tract infections.[5] It is possibly linked with cancer of the nose in workers who are exposed to high levels.

# Radon

Radon is a radioactive gas present to varying degrees in the soil, often in areas overlying igneous rock such as Cornwall, Devon and parts of Scotland, although it can also be present over shales, limestone and even alluvial soils. It is drawn into the house because air movement over the roof and around the walls produces a slight lowering of pressure relative to the gas pressure in the soil.

The levels of radon in the home can be assessed for £15–20 by asking the local authority to place a small pot in the house for about six weeks. If levels are high, they can be lowered by placing a small fan under the floor of the house, which draws out the gas before it filters into the house. New houses built in high-radon areas can be protected by a plastic membrane laid under the floor of the house.

Radon emits alpha particles, a kind of radiation that is particularly prone to causing cancer, and it is known that uranium miners have a high risk of lung cancer. It is sometimes the case that indoor levels are higher than those found in mines. Radon delivers about half of the radiation dose received by humans in the UK. If a smoker is exposed to radon, the risk of lung cancer is increased by a factor of ten. However, epidemiological studies do not yet show clearly what the risk is. Levels of radon are high in Scotland, and Scottish women have the highest lung cancer levels in the world but, on the other hand, levels of radon are also high in south-west England, and lung cancers there are low. Despite this discrepancy, the National Radiological Protection Board estimates that 1500 deaths from lung cancer annually are caused by radon.

A cost–benefit analysis of fitting protective device to homes is problematical.

Each year about 32 000 patients with lung cancer are treated, at a cost to the NHS of £85 million. The cost of radon-induced lung cancer may therefore be estimated at 4.6% of this, or £3 910 000. (There are, of course other social costs of the disease and its mortality.)

Against this, the cost of installing a 75-W extractor fan is as follows:

| | | |
|---|---|---|
| Unit cost | = | £100 |
| Installation cost | = | £100 |

If a unit lasts for ten years, then:
Annual installation cost = £20

Running cost = 75 W × 24 h × 365 days = 657 kWh @7.73p per kWh = £51

Therefore:
Total annual cost per home = £71.

No. homes to be fitted = 100 000–200 000
Total annual cost = £7 100 000–£14 200 000

If it takes two days' work to fit the fan, about 5000–10 000 job–years of work will be created, which will also carry general social and economic benefits. It may be that more extended analysis would make the figures more favourable, and of course people who are cancer phobic might be motivated to fit the device on a private basis if they live in high-radon homes.

Cornwall and Devon have been declared 'affected areas', which means that all home owners can have free radon measurements. Builders must put radon-proofing measures in place in the worst-affected areas.

# Perfumes

Clinical evidence exists that the strong odours of synthetic perfumes of the so-called 'air freshener' type may make people ill.[6,7] Since 1979, 89 cases have been found in a general practice in the West Country: an incidence of one case every two months on average. The syndrome is similar to hyperventilation syndrome, with feelings of unreality (derealization), anxiety, tearfulness, headaches and sleep disorder being the main features. There is usually unsteadiness on standing with feet together and eyes closed. Recovery follows two weeks after perfumes have been purged from the personal environment, including its removal from clothes which have been washed in powders claiming to be 'fresh'. Similar problems have been noted in the USA.[8] A study of young college students showed that two-thirds reported feeling ill on smelling a group of chemicals including perfume.[9] Further evidence is found in the fact that odorants are being used as therapeutic agents not only by aromatherapists, but also by workers with a scientific approach.[10] Basic pharmacological wisdom teaches that if a drug can have a positive effect, it almost certainly has a negative effect also.

There are sound neuroanatomical reasons for expecting over-strong stimulation of the brain's odour-sensing system to cause nervous problems, since the part of the brain that processes odour perception is now primarily occupied with dealing with emotions.

Nevertheless, these observations are just clinical anecdotes at present, serving to raise the hypothesis that the new, strong breed of synthetic perfumes can cause neuropsychological upset. The hypothesis needs to be tested. Unfortunately, we are faced with the impossibility of carrying out double-blind tests, in which one group of volunteers exposed to the odorants is compared with another who are not so exposed. Two wings of a jail might be used, one exposed to active air fresheners and one to dummies, but even so the subjects would not be 'blind', and neither would their assessors. Any trial carried out on these lines would therefore face criticism on the grounds that the experimental subjects would know that they were being exposed to odorants because their noses would tell them so.

Even so, it could be argued that any evidence would be better than none, and that an experiment should be carried out comparing two groups along the lines suggested above. There is a Consumer Safety Unit at the Department of Trade and Industry. The proposal that this would be a proper area to study was originally rejected on the grounds that, although on the face of it many thousands of people were at risk, none had died or been made seriously ill. A second obstacle was that no causal connection was established (R J Roscoe, Consumer Safety Unit, Department of Trade and Industry, personal communication, 27 September 1991) which is somewhat paradoxical, since the purpose of the investigation is to test the causality hypothesis. A further approach in March 1995 elicited the response that the Department of Health had not received any reports of adverse reactions to odorants. Clearly the Department of Trade and Industry had not passed the earlier report to the relevant department.

This is another example of official failure to understand the precautionary principle, and of the assumption that the onus of proof is on the victim of side-effects of commercial products to 'prove' that the product is harmful, when clearly they lack the considerable resources needed to do so. A third problem is that three government departments – Health, Trade and Industry and Environment – were involved, and therefore that effective action was unlikely to result.

Let us assume that there is a problem with these perfumes. If one GP sees six affected patients per year, and there are 30 000 GPs, this suggests an annual incidence of 180 000 people who are sufficiently affected by these perfumes to attend the doctor. This is the tip of an iceberg, because at least as many more will not attend but suffer on their own. If, of these 180 000, one in ten is offered tranquillizers and, of those, one in ten becomes addicted, and so continues to take them until death, we can make some estimates.

Cost of GP consultations: three per case @ £9.43  =  £5 092 200
Cost of Valium for two weeks for 18 000  =  £21 244

Cost of Valium for 30 years for 1800      =    £1 657 001

Total yearly cost of air fresheners      =    £6 770 445

Note that the 30-year cost is included in this year's costings, since it is the 'harvest' of this year's incidence. Next year a further harvest will be expected, so that the cost will be cumulative.

## Other pollutants

Volatile organic compounds (VOCs), mainly solvents from paints and plastics, accumulate in indoor air, as do a variety of breakdown products caused by the action of micro-organisms on plastics, especially foam carpet underlay.

## OUTDOOR AIR POLLUTION

Most forms of long-term low-dose outdoor air pollution also feature in indoor air pollution, since there is a constant slow exchange between the two types of air. Only coarse particulate pollution is significantly lower indoors than outdoors.

## General pollution and allergy

Studies have shown that general, mixed air pollution doubles the dose effectiveness of ragweed allergenicity and that, as general pollution increases, so too do the levels of IgE in the affected population.

## Ozone

Under certain atmospheric conditions caused by the action of sunlight on pollutants emitted from traffic, oxygen, $O_2$, can change into ozone, $O_3$. Photocopiers are a prolific source of ozone, and in poorly ventilated offices ozone levels can reach levels of 1000 $\mu g/m^3$. The levels in airliner cabins are high, although commercial airlines are not prepared to divulge a figure.

The triple formation of ozone is unstable, so that at the smallest excuse, the molecule reverts to $O_2$, releasing one highly reactive atom of oxygen – a 'free radical'. At a cellular level, ozone inhalation promotes inflammatory reactions in the airways, stimulates the release of cytokines (inflammatory messenger substances) and inhibits the action of macrophages (scavenger cells). All of this leads to damage of the epithelial cells that line the airways.

The effects of this on the individual are:

1 irritation of trachea, throat and eye
2 increased bronchial reactivity – that is there is a tendency to wheeze, which is the sign of asthma. Both asthmatics and non-asthmatics are affected in this way. Concentrations of ozone in the air show positive variation with hospital admissions for asthma – that is, when ozone is high, asthma admissions likewise are high
3 a possible carcinogenic effect. Free radicals in general are associated with cancer, and animal experimentation, regrettable although this is, has provided support. The US Department of Health National Toxicology Program showed that female mice exposed to high (2000 $\mu g/m^3$) levels of ozone for two years had a doubled risk of developing lung cancer. Male mice showed lesser effects and rats showed no effect. On the basis of this evidence the Americans and Germans, siding with the mice, have decided to classify ozone as a possible carcinogen, whereas the British Health and Safety Executive (HSE) has chosen to assume that the British people are more like rats, and have decided to abolish the 200 $\mu g/m^3$ limit for ozone at work.

The World Health Organization's safety limit is 100 $\mu g/m^3$. Levels of up to 240 $\mu g/m^3$ are commonly registered in outdoor air in summer.

## Sulphur dioxide

High levels of sulphur dioxide in the air causes wheezing in asthmatics, and long-term exposure is associated with chronic bronchitis. It seems logical that sulphur dioxide cannot be associated with asthma since sulphur dioxide levels have been falling while asthma levels have been rising. However, even this simple fact is not clear in the intensely complicated field of pollution science. Three papers[11,12,13] suggest that long-term exposure to sulphur dioxide may increase the prevalence of bronchial hyperresponsiveness (BHR), which is a measure of the irritability of the airways. It is not the same thing as asthma, being a more precise, measurable estimation, but acts as a proxy for asthma in a population. In a study of two Norwegian valleys,[14] fluoride accompanied the sulphur dioxide as a pollutant, which may have been a confounding factor.

## Volatile organic compounds

Many compounds come under this heading, but benzene is one of the most important to human health. It is a genotoxic carcinogen, and is under suspicion of being a co-factor in the causation of leukaemia, as well as lung, kidney, pancreas and stomach cancer. Petrol pump attendants are the 'critical group', that is the group most at risk, although those living near petrol stations are also exposed to significant doses. Seventy-eight per cent of benzene in the air comes from petrol engines, and 'super unleaded' petrol is the most prolific source of benzene.

1,3-Butadeine is another genotoxic carcinogen that is present in petrol and exhaust fumes.

Occupational exposure to petrol and diesel fuels is associated with increased risk of a variety of cancers.

## Nitrogen dioxide

Road vehicles produce more than 50% of the nitrogen oxides found in outdoor air. The gas is known to slow the action of the cilia, the respiratory tract's self-cleaning mechanism. The levels of nitrogen dioxide in air have been found to be proportional to respiratory disease admissions to hospital at concentrations less than 154 ppb. Levels may be proportional to admissions to hospital for croup. It is not yet certain whether this is a direct effect of nitrogen dioxide or whether the nitrogen dioxide level is merely acting as an indicator for general pollution.

## Fine particles

Interest has recently been focused on the disease-provoking effects of fine particles which are less than ten microns in diameter (PM10s), and even more on those that are less than 2.5 microns in diameter. Their tiny size means that they penetrate far deeper into the lungs than larger smoke particles. It is possible that PM10s derived from diesel may have different properties from those derived from petrol.

Road vehicles produce 70% of PM10s in the atmosphere. In the USA, a study of the population of six cities has shown that the level of PM10s in the air is proportional to mortality from heart disease, lung disease and cancer.[15] It has been found that a 100 $\mu g/m^3$ rise in the particles will result in a 16% increase in mortality rate. The most polluted cities had a 26% higher overall death rate and a 37% higher cardiopulmonary death rate than the least polluted.

Levels of PM10s are proportional to rates of asthma episodes, chest disease and school absences.

## Asbestos

Heavy goods vehicle brakepads still contain asbestos. Each time the brakes are applied, tiny amounts of asbestos are released into the air, adding to the lung cancer risk of the general population. This is another reason for sending freight by rail.

## Industrial air pollution

It is not easy to quantify at national level the health effects of air pollution experienced by populations living in the lee of industrial plant. There is a vast literature of studies of individual sites, but by no means all sites have been covered. The effect will depend on the nature of the emissions and the nature of the population. The one constant factor will be that the population affected will tend to be less affluent than average, since the wealthier citizens will long since have moved out, so the health effects of deprivation have a confounding influence on any studies. The emission aspect of the problem has two components:

1   the nature of the emissions, and
2   the pattern of the fallout.

Fallout pattern is a rather neglected aspect of air pollution. Studies that simply compare health statistics of populations grouped according to their proximity to the emission source are open to question, since the important feature is the 'plume' of pollution, that is its pattern of deposition on the ground. People living close to the plant upwind may receive a lower dose than those further away downwind, and specific topographic features may result in high levels of pollution at certain points for a given wind direction.

Under the old 'dilute and disperse' philosophy of industrial waste management, it was thought to be sufficient to build a tall chimney to stop the immediate neighbourhood from choking within a week of the plant's opening. As the clouds of ignorance have slowly dispersed, it has been seen that tall chimneys only transfer the problem somewhere else and make the effects more difficult to distinguish. The key assumption of 'dilute and disperse' is that the pollutants are evenly mixed in the air mass through turbulence. In fact, this does not happen in four common meteorological conditions: inversion, anticyclones, thermal formation and specific microclimatic conditions.

Inversion occurs when blocks of warm air lie on top of layers of cool air, as when warm air masses are pushed north and also when cold and warm fronts coincide. A bowl-like local topography will amplify the effects of an inversion. By their nature inversions are stable, and may persist for several days. Any pollutants released in the air will not be diluted or dispersed, but stay right in the locality, producing progressively poorer air quality.

Anticyclonic conditions – still, settled air, as on fine summer days – may also create the same non-dispersal conditions.

Thermals are at the other end of the weather spectrum, occurring when warm air lies under cooler layers. Bubbles of warm air, whose size varies from a few hundred feet to thousands of feet in diameter, break from the ground and rise until they cool sufficiently to form cumulus clouds – best seen as the white puffy clouds of spring, deeply beloved by gliders and hang-gliders for their antigravity properties, and equally disliked by some air travellers as the cause of bumpiness.

Any pollution released at the point that a thermal breaks from the ground – which may be many times a day in good conditions – will find itself encapsulated in its own cumulus cloud. If and when the contents of the clouds are dropped as a shower, the packet of pollution will be deposited as a 'hotspot'. Such deposits are impossible to predict, but may have small health effects on the receiving population.

Local topography and microclimate may affect the dispersal of emissions. Wind passing over a factory will travel in specific paths, skipping over some areas and coming down on to the surface in other areas. More attention should be paid to these atmospheric features in the study and regulation of industrial pollution.

If local people suspect that their health is being put at risk by air emissions from local industrial plant, they should contact the environmental health department of their local authority. If the plant is a 'Part A' process, that is a major industry, the complaint will be passed on to the Pollution Inspectorate. Both environmental health officers and pollution inspectors are empowered to investigate the problem and to require the process to be cleaned up, but it must be admitted that in the majority of cases the initial assumption on the part of the officers is that the emissions are innocent until proved guilty. Officers rely heavily on the voluntary cooperation of the industry; they are reluctant to bear down heavily on people with whom they must work regularly. The industry's scientists will often be more *au fait* with the details of the process than the investigators, and better prepared for a detailed debate. The outcome of the complaint depends very much on local condition, the workload, disposition and political leadership of the local environmental health team being key factors. Environmental health officers are highly trained, competent and professional people, but like doctors they are not infallible. Citizens may find that the scholastic method – 'the book says that no health effects are to be expected, therefore there are none' – is being employed rather than the scientific: 'how can we test the hypothesis that the emissions are causing ill health?'. For these reasons, it is sometimes necessary for local people to form a campaign group with all the trappings of publicity in order to motivate the officers. Untrained locals, aided perhaps by environmentalists and sympathetic professionals, will find themselves working unpaid in their spare time, ranged against professionals who are well paid to deal with these matters throughout their professional lives. It is a testimony to the resourcefulness and motivation of local people that in the end they are often victorious.

Even if evidence of ill-health is found, British law has another card up its sleeve to confound the victim. Case law cannot take into account the particular sensitivity of the individual. This means that the health effect should be found in everyone, or at least the majority of those exposed to the emission. In particular, allergic reactions, even life-threatening anaphylaxis and crippling extrinsic alveolitis, are excluded from consideration. There is clearly a need for this aspect of law to be reformed.

An alternative is to use Section 8 of the Environmental Protection Act, which allows controls to be brought on any emission which is 'prejudicial to health'. Because of the relative newness of the Act, this has not yet been tested in court.

Some of the most important pollutants emitted by industry are described in the book *Air Quality Guideliness for Europe*[16], which lists other air pollutants that are of importance to human health – acrylonitrile, carbon disulphide,

1,2-dichlorethane, dichloromethane, polyaromatic hydrocarbons, styrene, tetra-chlorethylene, toluene, trichloroethylene, vinyl chloride and about ten inorganic substances. Most are suspected or known to have carcinogenic or central nervous system effects. The World Health Organization and the EU set standards for their concentration in air that will limit them to subtoxic levels, but our knowledge of their effects in combination with each other or with other pollutants in the home in certain vulnerable people is not so complete that effects occurring at legal levels can be ruled out.

Although it is not possible to quantify the effects of industry on populations with any degree of accuracy, there must be health effects, and these effects will neces-sarily be reflected in NHS expenditure. In order to form a rough estimate and rep-resentation of these costs, let us use the 1990 Environmental Protection Act Part 1, which sets out processes to be controlled by the Pollution Inspectorate (1800 major processes) and those to be controlled by local authorities (27 000 minor processes). Let us assume that 1000 people live in the lee of each Part A process, and assign a £10 increase in NHS expenditure for each person. Let us further assume that 500 people are affected by Part B processes, and that the extra cost is £5.

$$
\begin{array}{lll}
\text{Part A processes: } 1800 \times 1000 \times \pounds10 & = & \pounds18\ 000\ 000 \\
\text{Part B processes: } 27\ 000 \times 500 \times 5 & = & \pounds67\ 500\ 000 \\
\\
\text{Total estimated cost to NHS} & = & \pounds85\ 500\ 000 \text{ per year}
\end{array}
$$

It might be argued that the trend in this kind of illness has been decreasing over the last two decades owing to the general rundown of UK manufacturing industry. How-ever, since emissions of any kind represent a waste of actual or potential resources, and since techniques and technology exist to bring emissions down to near zero, and since curbing emissions can actually make an installation more profitable, it may be argued that all of the above estimated expenditure is unnecessary.

# DRINKING WATER

## Drinking water: quantity

Like shelter and warmth, clean water is a basic necessity for life, and in a civilized country should be available to all. This is not to say that it should be available free of charge, since water is a scarce resource, even in the relatively rainy climate of the UK, and much energy and human work is necessary to bring it from rainfall to consumer. In the south of England water is in short supply and is being abstracted from underground sources at such a rate that river levels are sometimes affected. It is our duty to conserve water supplies and not to treat it as an infinite resource freely available at all times for non-essential purposes such as washing cars; but

**Table 9.1**  Use of domestic water

| Purpose | Water use (%) |
|---|---|
| Drinking | 2.5 |
| Gardening and outside | 3 |
| Washing machine | 12 |
| Washing, baths, showers | 17 |
| WC flushing, waste disposal | 32 |
| Mains leakage (+dripping taps and car washing) | 33.5 |

this need to conserve ought not to affect the supply of water as a basic necessity of life for all. Surprisingly, one of the main causes of water wastage is leakage from ageing mains supplies. Table 9.1 shows the use of domestic water.

The source of Table 9.1 is the Water Companies Association. Credit for ingenuity must be given for conflating mains leakage with dripping taps and car washing. Although dripping taps and car washing are clearly wasteful activities, they can hardly amount to more than 5% of the total: but they have been used to divert attention from the fact that about 30% of pure water is lost from mains leakage. Clearly, there is scope for use of the privatized water companies' handsome profits in an intensive investment in new mains. Work for this programme could attract wage subsidy support.

In view of this centralized wastage, it seems even more unacceptable that people who are unable to pay their water bills should be cut off. The recent privatization of water has turned out to mean that the universal availability of drinking water on tap to everyone can no longer be assumed. Water prices have risen by 50% since privatization. In 1992, 21 000 households were disconnected while the water companies announced pre-tax profits of £1.5 billion, and in 1994 nearly 2 million households defaulted on their water bills. The number of houses in water debt is nine times greater now than when water privatization was introduced in 1989.[17] As might be expected, the brunt of debt falls on the unemployed family in council rented housing in an area with high water bills.

There is no code of practice to advise water companies as to when disconnection might be inappropriate, as is the case with the electricity and gas companies. In Scotland disconnection is not allowed, and a spirited political opposition of the Scottish people prevented privatization itself.

Clearly, a household that is disconnected will be unable to maintain standards of hygiene, which carries with it the risk of transmitting infectious diseases, especially those that are transmitted by the faecal–oral route. This being so, we should expect to find an increase in this kind of disease in poor areas following privatization. The figures are consistent with this expectation (Table 9.2).

The 1991 level was the highest level of dysentery for 20 years, and carried a cost to the public sector of £1 175 288.

Outbreaks of hepatitis A have occurred among communities with high rates of water disconnection.

**Table 9.2** Trends in dysentery and hepatitis notifications

| Year | Dysentery cases | Hepatitis A cases |
| --- | --- | --- |
| 1987 | – | 1126 |
| 1989 | 2011 | 3431 |
| 1990 | 1489 | – |
| 1991 | 8071 | 5610 |

These increases cannot be assumed to be due to disconnection alone, but they are likely to play a part. (In any case, the precise cause is not relevant for the purposes of assessing the burden that the increases throw on the NHS.) The way to determine how large a part is to remove disconnection as an option for water companies, to restore supplies to disconnected households and to observe what, if any, difference this makes to the figures for hygiene-related conditions.

## Recommendation

That water companies should be given protocols to control the circumstances of people who fail to pay their water rates, short of disconnection.

# Drinking water quality

## Microbial contamination

Three-quarters of the citizens of a rural Irish town whose water supply became exposed to sewage became ill, with symptoms including abdominal cramps, diarrhoea, loss of appetite, nausea and tiredness.[18] The interesting aspect of this is that no pathogen was found in the faeces of affected people, so either a hitherto unrecognized pathogen was at work or the illness was a general reaction to the challenge of contaminated water. Given the decrepit state of many of our ageing sewers and water mains, which often lie close to each other, contamination may often go unrecognized. Normally the high pressure in the water main keeps sewage out, but drops in pressure due to high demand and/or supply problems may allow ingress of foul water into drinking water supplies.

*Cryptosporidium* is an organism that occasionally contaminates drinking water. It is difficult to eradicate as it is resistant to chlorination. It causes outbreaks of diarrhoea, abdominal cramps and fever that may last up to three weeks, and is very much worse in AIDS sufferers. There was an outbreak in 1989 in Swindon.

## Chlorine

Chlorine is added to drinking water in order to sterilize it: without chlorine, intestinal infections would be rife. All British water is chlorinated, but in the USA chlorine is often not added to water extracted from deep aquifers and distributed through modern pipes. American epidemiologists therefore have access to a group that is not exposed to chlorine, which enables them to make health comparisons with populations in chlorinated areas. The results are very interesting.

American researchers carried out a meta-analysis (that is a summation of all the respectable research that they could find) on chlorine.[19] They found that the relative risk of cancer in people exposed to chlorinated water was 1.15 (that is a 15% increase over normal). In particular, they found a 21% increase for bladder cancer and 38% increase for rectal cancer.

This increase is not surprising. Chlorine has an oxidative effect, and can be expected to produce free radicals in the body, which are associated with cancer causation.

Dutch researchers in a small pilot study[20] found chloroform in tiny amounts in the blood of competitive swimmers in an indoor pool. They found evidence of renal damage in the younger swimmers. This was a small pilot study which needs to be repeated with larger numbers.

For the purposes of costing, let us assume that the chlorination of Britain's water supply is responsible for 1% of all cancers. Taking the 1991 cost of neoplasms to the NHS of £923 million, we have a chlorine-generated cost of £9.23 million per year.

Could these costs be avoided? Simply to stop putting chlorine in the drinking water is not an option, since it would result in increased infections from contaminated drinking water, but there are alternative water-sterilizing methods. Ozone can be used instead of chlorine, but it lacks the long-term sterilizing properties of chlorine. Ultraviolet light is effective, but only at the point where it is applied. Micro-organisms can survive in shade under flakes of rust and further down the pipe where the light does not reach. A new and elegant method of sterilization passes water between copper and silver electrodes. Tiny amounts of ionized metals pass into the water, killing bacteria and algae. The drawback is that the metals are lost irrevocably: they cannot be re-used or recycled, so that in the long term it would be impractical to use the process on all water. However, for some applications, this method is useful, for example in swimming baths, avoiding the irritant and unhealthy effects of chlorine, and in large institutions, to protect against the danger of contamination of the water supply with *Legionella*.

In general, therefore, the only alternative is to remove the chlorine at the 'pipe end' by using activated charcoal or other water filters. All filters from the jug type to the varieties of plumbed-in filters will perform this basic and very important function. Although 'pipe end' removal is usually seen as a second best alternative to avoiding contamination in the first place, in this case the approach is reasonable since the filter also removes many other unwanted contaminants.

All filters need to be changed regularly to avoid becoming ineffective or even infected. The initial cost of fitting filters to all of Britain's 22 million households would come to £2.2 billion, with an additional yearly cost of £1.1 billion to renew the filters. This would seem prohibitive, and it is likely that if it were to be performed as public service the expenditure would in the main be wasted as under-motivated and impoverished households would fail to renew the filters because of the trouble and expense involved. Filters which are neglected may become infected and hazardous. So it is likely that filtration of water will continue to be carried out on a private basis, and will grow as more people become aware of the dangers of drinking chlorine (and the other contaminants in drinking water) and of the taste advantages of making tea with chlorine-free water. (Chlorine combines with phenols in rubber fittings in the kettle to produce the TCP taste that is often noticeable in tea.) This situation is far from ideal since it leads again to a widening of the health gap between rich and poor. Filters would be cheaper if filter companies were eligible for the wage subsidy and tax breaks.

Another hazard of chlorination is that of inhalation of chlorine by-products, notably trihalomethanes, from hot water, especially showers. The effects of trihalomethanes are carcinogenicity and liver damage. This exposure can be avoided by fitting a charcoal filter to the pipe leading to the shower or bath.

## Lead

Lead reaches us via drinking water, air (from leaded petrol), dust (from leaded petrol), food (from leaded petrol and from lead solder in cans) and paint (high levels are available in British paint, although other countries have legislated for safety levels). Its effect is to lower intelligence. Maybe Britons are caught in a vicious circle.

Lead piping is still fitted in some areas, and dissolved lead is a particular problem in soft water areas. In 1976 7% of British homes exceeded the then EU limit of 100 μg/l for lead in drinking water: in Scotland the figure was 34%. Since then the safety levels have been revised downwards: the 'flushed' (that is, after the water has run to get rid of lead dissolved into the pipe while the tap was not being used) level was changed to 50 μg/l, then to 30 μg/l, and the level for infants' bottle feed is now 10–15 μg/l. In practical terms, this is tantamount to saying that, if there is lead piping in the house, water for infants feeds should be filtered.

Grants are available to assist households in replacing lead piping (water companies will not replace pipes within the curtilage of a house) but the programme is proceeding at a snail's pace.

The main effect of lead at the levels expected in water will be to reduce intelligence of the affected population by one or two IQ points for a doubling in the body burden of lead,[21] and possibly to add to the behaviour disorders of children.

At higher levels of ingestion, for example caused by a child eating old lead paint, stomach pains, headaches, tremor, irritability, coma and death may result.

It is almost impossible to quantify the cost to society and the NHS of the effects of lead plumbing, but it is certain that they will continue as long as the house is in use. The replacement of the pipes should therefore be seen as a long-term investment in the health of future generations, as well as a useful provision of work for today's unemployed.

The time required for replacing lead piping is 0.5–2 days, at a (1994) cost of about £130 – less if wage subsidy and VAT exemption are applied. Assuming a one-day average job time, to complete the work on 7% of Britain's housing stock would create about 4000 job–years of work.

In order to register the cost of lead poisoning to the NHS, a value of 0.001% of the 1991 NHS spend on mental disorders (£2724 million) will be taken, i.e. £2.7 million.

## Aluminium

Aluminium is deliberately added to water by water companies as a flocculant in order to clarify it – about 100 000 tonnes are added per year. Normally, much of this is removed before reaching the mains, but if controls are imperfect some will find its way into drinking water. Acid rain will add to this by dissolving aluminium from rocks into water. It is also deliberately added to water by consumers as tea, which contains high levels of aluminium. Aluminium cooking pots add to the burden and, finally, we consume huge quantities in the form of antacid medicines.

A cloud of suspicion hangs over aluminium because it is found in the neurofibrillary tangles in the brains of Alzheimer's disease sufferers, and because renal dialysis patients, who take in large amounts of aluminium, sometimes develop a form of dementia. Does the aluminium help to cause the disease or does it merely get itself attached to the tangles after they have formed, by accident?

The evidence that aluminium is involved in causation is pretty damning. The incidence of Alzheimer's has been shown several times to be higher in areas where there is more aluminium in the water. Treatment with chelating drugs, which remove metals from the body, slows the progress of Alzheimer's.[22]

The deposition of aluminium has been shown to be very precisely within the tangles rather than applied to the outside like barnacles on a ship's bottom.[23] It would not be correct to say that aluminium is the only cause of Alzheimer's; genetic factors and other dietary factors (essential fatty acids) may well be involved, but the precautionary principle clearly calls for a reduction in deliberate introduction of aluminium in our water.

There is also some evidence that aluminium contributes to hyperactivity and learning difficulties in children,[24] and to bone disease.

---

### Recommendations

1  That aluminium as a flocculant should be phased out as soon as possible and iron salts used as flocculants for drinking water if this is thought necessary.

2  That aluminium cooking utensils and aluminium-containing antacids are either banned or highly taxed, with the taxes hypothecated to research and treatment of Alzheimer's disease.

3  That an extra tax be introduced on tea and other high-aluminium foods, to be hypothecated to the care of Alzheimer's sufferers in proportion to the best estimate of the contribution to the problem made by the foodstuffs.

Cost: a notional cost of 0.001% of the NHS cost of mental services will be taken: £2.7 million per year.

## Nitrate

High levels of nitrate in drinking water are associated with a rare condition of babies called methaemoglobinaemia. Bottle-fed infants under nine months are at risk if the level of nitrate exceeds 50 mg/l. The last death from this condition was in 1948.

There is a suspicion that nitrates in drinking water may be associated with cancer of the stomach. Nitrates may turn into nitrites and then carcinogenic nitrosamines. However, epidemiological studies to date have not linked high levels of nitrate in drinking water with increased rates of stomach cancer.

## Pesticides

These are often present in low levels in drinking water, and the EU guidelines are not infrequently breached. The significance of this will be covered in chapter 10.

# RIVER AND SEAWATER

Twenty per cent of Britain's beaches failed the EU Bathing Water Directive in 1994. In 1995 that figure will increase to 30% as more stringent rules are introduced. The UK dumps 300 million gallons of raw sewage into the sea every day. In Denmark all beaches pass, because no Danish sewage is disposed of to sea, it is all treated and recycled to land where it completes the natural cycle: plants nourish us, and our waste nourishes the plants. To be safely returned to land, sewage sludge must be free of industrial contaminants, biologically digested and pasteurized to kill viruses. The liquid effluent can be sterilized by exposure to ultraviolet radiation in the form of natural sunlight in lagoons, or passed under UV lights. This technology is not difficult. The difficulty is in the lack of political will, in that public investment in these improvements for the sake of public and environmental health is required. The free market, like its polar opposite, the command economies of the old USSR, is incapable of delivering this kind of environmental improvement.

Given our propensity for bathing in a dilute solution of our own wastes, it is not surprising that some of us become infected from time to time.

Evidence is mounting of the health risks from bathing in polluted seawater. Several studies have confirmed that illnesses such as sore throat, conjunctivitis and gastroenteritis may result from bathing, especially if the head is immersed. The best designed of these studies took place in the UK in 1989,[25] wherein 1000 volunteers were divided into two groups. Half took a ten-minute dip on one of four beaches which had passed on the EU standards, while the other half just stayed on the beach. Table 9.3 shows some of the results.

Bacteria do not survive as long in seawater as viruses, and fewer viruses are required to start an infection than bacteria. The spirit of EU regulations requires

**Table 9.3**  The risks of bathing in contaminated seawater[25]

| Illness | Relative risk factor |
| --- | --- |
| Sore throat | 2–3 |
| Eye infection | 8 |
| Cough | 3 |
| Abdominal pain | 2 |
| Loose motions | 2 |
| 'Flu-like illness | 2 |
| Respiratory illness | 1.8 |

A relative risk factor of two would mean that a swimmer is twice as likely to get that illness as the average person.

that viruses should be monitored, but this is not often done because the tests are more expensive than for bacteria. In the past it has been argued that bacterial levels will indicate to what degree viruses are present, but this has been shown not to be so. The astrovirus, which can cause gastroenteritis, has been identified on British bathing beaches in quantities that are more than enough to cause illness.

More worryingly, hepatitis A can be caught from seawater, and also from eating inadequately cooked shellfish brought up from contaminated waters. As they are filter feeders, shellfish concentrate the virus. It is suspected that viral meningitis may also be transmitted via seawater.

It is known that poliomyelitis can be transmitted via infected water, but received opinion is that it is not caused by sewage pollution in seawater because dilutions are so great and because most of the community is immune. Most polioviruses found now in sewage are derived from live polio vaccine, which 'do not commonly cause severe permanent nerve disease' – a delicate way of saying that they may cause temporary and incomplete paralysis.

# Eutrophication

This condition occurs when any body of water is sufficiently contaminated with phosphates from sewage. Algae may grow abundantly in these fertile waters to the detriment of other species. Dead algae sink to the bottom, and their decay uses up oxygen so that other life forms die. In freshwater, blue–green algae blooms can be a threat to anything that comes into contact with the water. They are quite common in any lake or reservoir which receives farm runoff. In Blagdon Lake, a reservoir in north-west Somerset, the presence of blue–green algae is taken as routine in the summer months. It makes the fish drowsy and lethargic, and may poison dogs which swim in the water. Canoeists have been affected on at least one occasion. The algae's neurotoxin is thought to be removed during the treatment process that prepares the water for human consumption. It would be better all round, including economically, to treat the farmyard waste in such a way that the watercourses are not contaminated with a valuable fertilizer.

Seawater is affected by algal blooms as a result of the dumping of sewage or sewage sludge at sea. Some species may produce neurotoxins, although none is known to affect humans.

## Sewage treatment

The first stage in sewage treatment is screening to remove items such as wood, cloth or plastics. This is followed by settling out of solids. Regrettably, solids may still be dumped at sea, in landfill, or incinerated. This not only causes environmental pollution, but also represents a wasted resource. The preferred treatment is anaerobic digestion (or other forms of digestion that are becoming available) and return to agricultural or forestry land. Return to land requires that industrial waste containing toxic substances is not mixed in with domestic sewage. Anaerobic digestion has the triple virtues of:

1  producing a methane-rich gas which can be used for heating or driving cars
2  producing a fertilizer which is particularly valuable for conditioning soils damaged by industrial farming
3  killing off bacterial pathogens. The sludge must be pasteurized to kill off viruses which survive the anaerobic process.

The liquid left after separation still has a heavy biological oxygen demand. If released into rivers it would absorb all the oxygen and cause fish to be killed. It is therefore mixed with air by a variety of means. The organisms active in this treatment also reduce some of the pathogens in the liquid.

Chlorination is sometimes used to sterilize minced whole sewage or inadequately treated liquid effluent before it is stupidly piped into the sea. The chlorine can have adverse effects on the ecology of the watercourse. Better than chlorination is to use ultraviolet light to sterilize the effluent or to pass it through reed beds.

## LANDFILLS AND CONTAMINATED LAND

Ordinary landfill sites pollute groundwater[26] and air. Leaching of rainwater through the site and into the ground is inevitable even in those lined with a membrane and placed on clay, since their capacity to absorb rainwater is limited; some is bound to spill over. The leachate from landfill sites is similar in composition to liquid sewage spiced with heavy metals. The further a landfill is from an aquifer which is used for drinking water, the longer the contamination will take to reach the water supply, but contamination is in the end unavoidable. At very least, our landfills are forcing succeeding generations to incur costs in cleaning up drinking water supplies drawn from aquifers. It may even deny them the use of some sources of groundwater completely.

Seagulls may introduce *Clostridium botulinum* bacteria, which then multiply in the warm putrescible waste and reinfect the seagulls, with the resulting danger of introducing the bacterium into human food.[27]

The action of bacteria on putrescible wastes in landfill produces landfill gas, a mixture of methane, carbon dioxide and carbon monoxide. This gas is produced in quantity, and can migrate away from the site. In 1986, gas from a site at Loscoe, Derbyshire, collected in a basement distant from the site and ignited, destroying the house. People living in houses that have been built over landfill sites have complained of general poor health with headaches and tiredness predominating. Just because a landfill site has been designated for domestic waste does not necessarily mean that no hazardous waste has been dumped there by unscrupulous operators.

Old chemical works, gasworks, manufacturing sites and dumping ground pose an uncertain threat to human and environmental health. Records are incomplete, whereas sites are numerous: in Cheshire there are 1577 sites. *Caveat emptor* – if you buy a piece of land that turns out to be contaminated, the cost of the task of restoring it comes to you.

## Hazardous waste

Surprisingly little work has been done on the health hazards associated with hazardous (toxic) waste dumps. It is extremely difficult to establish direct causal links between hazardous waste and local people.[28]

The work that has been done has concentrated on the workforce, which numbers about 100 000 in the UK. Even this work is plagued with scientific difficulties since the waste is by definition mixed, which is anathema to non-system scientists who seek to discover a clear one-to-one relationship between one toxin and one effect. In addition, it is difficult to establish levels of exposure. In one study[29] it was impossible to distinguish in blood tests between those with high or low exposure. Gustavsson[30] examined the records of 176 workers who had dealt with hazardous waste, mainly heavy metals, and found an increase in lung cancer and ischaemic heart disease.

For populations living near hazardous waste sites, the main exposure route is from air-borne dusts and incinerator fallout. In the USA, houses were built over the old Love Canal toxic waste tip, and gases from the tip percolated into the indoor air.[31] The people so exposed complained of a variety of vague illnesses that do not fit into a diagnostic category, such as headaches, tiredness, and dizziness – complaints which can easily be dismissed by a sceptical official as nervous in origin, as was the case in Camelford.

Dumping is a second-rate way of managing waste. The rational approach:

1   avoids producing waste at source by assessing and amending processes
2   recycles waste within the process by purification and separation
3   treats waste in specific chemical reactions or innovative electrical, photochemi-
    cal processes which will degrade or separate it
4   uses biological methods, either digestion with micro-organisms or uptake into
    specific species of plant
5   applies state-of-the art dust and gas extraction to the chimney if incineration is
    used.

It will be seen that there is a great opportunity for growth in the waste management industry. This section of the economy should be supported with tax breaks
and wage subsidy.

# CONCLUSION

The growth of any biological species, including humans, is limited by space, nutrients and negative feedback from its own waste products. Our wastes are everywhere, which makes it difficult for us to assess their health effect because we
have no easily accessible comparator group. The health effects are in some cases
serious or lethal, but mostly a multiplicity of small, long-term influences whose
combined effect on human health we have not really begun to assess.

# REFERENCES

1   Dubos R (1970) *So Human an Animal.* Abacus, London.

2   Economics and Operational Research Division (1992) *Effect of Tobacco Advertising on
    Tobacco Consumption.* Department of Health, London.

3   Tobacco Advertising Bans Work. Action on Smoking and Health. Telephone: 0171
    935 5519.

4   Centre for Health Economics (1995) *Tobacco and Jobs.* Centre for Health Economics,
    University of York, York.

5   Hekwig H (1977) How safe is formaldehyde? *Deutsche Medizinische Wochenschrifte:*
    **102**; 1612–13.

6   Lawson R H (1985) Is there an air freshener syndrome? *Bristol Med Chir J:* **100**;
    10–13.

7   Lawson R H (1992) Air Freshener Perfumes. *Pyschiatric Bull:* **16**; 173.

8    Kendall J (1992) Citizens for a Toxic Free World. Indoor Air Quality as an Environmental Issue. *The New Reactor*: **1(10)**; 3.

9    Bell I R, Schwartz G E, Peterson J M *et al.* (1993) Self-reported illness from chemical odours in young adults without clinical syndromes of occupational exposure. *Arch Environ Health*: **48(1)**; 6–13.

10   Dodd G and Van Toller S (1993) *Perfumer and Flavourist*: **8**; 4.

11   Sheppard D (1988) Sulfur dioxide and asthma – a double-edged sword. *J Allergy Clin Immunol*: **82**; 961–4.

12   Ferris B G, Ware J H, Spengler J D (1988) Exposure measurement for air pollution epidemiology. In: L Gordis and C H Libauer (eds) *Epidemiology and Health Risk Assessment*. Oxford University Press, Oxford, pp. 120–7.

13   Andrae S, Axelson O, Bjorksten B *et al.* (1988) Symptoms of bronchial hyperreactivity in asthma in relation to environmental factors. *Arch Dis Child*: **63**; 473–8.

14   Soyseth V, Kongerud J, Harr D *et al.* (1995) Relation of exposure to airway irritants in infancy to prevalence of bronchial hyperresponsiveness in schoolchildren. *Lancet*: **345**; 217–20.

15   Dockery D W, Pope C C, Xu X *et al.* (1993) An association between air pollution and mortality in six US cities. *N Eng J Med*: **329**; 1753–9.

16   Turck R (1987) *Air Quality Guidelines for Europe*. WHO Publications, Copenhagen.

17   Policy Studies Institute (1995) *Water Debt and Disconnection*. Policy Studies Institute, London.

18   Fogarty J, Thornton L, Hayes C *et al.* (1995) Illness in a community associated with an episode of water contamination with sewage. *Epidemiol Infect*: **114(2)**; 289–95.

19   Morris R D, Audet A M, Angelillo I F *et al.* (1992) Chlorination, chlorination by-products, and cancer: a meta-analysis. *Am J Public Health*: **82**; 955–63.

20   Aiking H, van Acker M B, Scholten R J *et al.* (1994) Swimming pool chlorination: a health hazard? *Toxicol Lett*: **72**; 375–80.

21   Pocock S J, Smith M, Baghurst P (1994) Environmental lead and children's intelligence: a systematic review of the epidemiological evidence. *BMJ*: **309**; 1189–97.

22   McLachlan D R, Fraser P E, Dalton A J (1992) Aluminium and the pathogenesis of Alzheimer's disease: a summary of evidence. *Ciba Found Symp*: **169**; 87–98.

23   Perl D P and Good P F (1992) Aluminium and the neurofibrillary tangle: results of tissue microprobe studies. *Ciba Found Symp*: **169**; 217–27.

24   Cooke K and Gould M H (1991) The health effects of aluminium – a review. *J R Soc Health*: **111**; 163–8.

25   Balarajan R, Soni Raleigh V, Yuen P *et al.* (1991) Health risks associated with bathing in seawater. *BMJ*: **303**; 1444–5.

26   Croft B and Campbell D (1990) Characteristics of 100 UK landfill sites. In: *Proceedings of 1990 Harwell Waste Management Symposium*. UKAEA, Harwell.

**27**  Ortiz N E and Smith G R (1994) Landfill sites, botulism and gulls. *Epidemiol Infect*. **112**; 385–91.

**28**  Najem G R and Cappadona J L (1991) Health effects of hazardous chemical waste disposal sites in New Jersey and the United States: a review. *Am J Prevent Med*. **7**; 352–62.

**29**  Favata E A and Gochfield M (1989) Medical surveillance of hazardous waste workers: ability of laboratory tests to discriminate exposure. *Am J Ind Med*. **15**; 255–65.

**30**  Gustavsson P (1989) Mortality among workers at a municipal waste incinerator. *Am J Ind Med*. **15**; 245–53.

**31**  Paigen B *et al.* (1984) Prevalence of health problems in children living near Love Canal. *J Am Med Assoc*. **251**; 1437–40.

# 10

# Food and drugs

*Them belly full but we hungry*
*A hungry man is an angry man*

Bob Marley

## INTRODUCTION

There is a resistible temptation to begin any discussion of food with the cliché 'you are what you eat'. We are more than what we eat, just as a home is more than bricks and mortar, but it is true that diet is of immense importance to our health, and that there is evidence that in some ways our diet is deteriorating. This chapter cannot hope to cover the subject comprehensively, but will pick out some of the current issues and controversies, with an eye on what government can do to improve the situation.[1]

## QUANTITY

It is a sad reflection on the rationality of human economics and our sense of equity that, whereas obesity due to overeating is a problem in the nations of the north, food scarcity is the problem in the south, and that some sections of our own society go short of the basic human freedom, the freedom from hunger. The scandal is all the greater because it has been estimated by some that 30% of food bought in shops is wasted. An Office of Health Economics report[2] calculates the direct cost of obesity to the NHS at £29.35 million per year, and the indirect costs in contributing to heart attacks, stroke, late-onset diabetes mellitus, osteoarthritis and hypertension at £165.25 million – a total of £194.60 million. The report took a conservative estimate of the contribution obesity made to the indirect costs. A higher estimate was made in The Netherlands, where a study[3] concluded that obesity-related conditions absorbed 6% of the Dutch health budget each year. Importing this figure to the NHS budget gives a figure of £2 billion per year. Since obesity has doubled in ten years, it follows that the NHS has become relatively poorer to the tune of between £100 and £1000 million per year over the course of the last ten years.

---

### Recommendation

Government action on obesity should include a sugar tax and cycleway provision.

---

# QUALITY

The balanced diet consists of:

- proteins
- carbohydrates
- fats, including essential fatty acids
- fibre
- minerals
- vitamins
- not too many toxins.

All too often the diet we eat now consists of sugar, fats, more sugar, additives, protein, *trans* fats, additives, more sugar and not enough fibre, vitamins or minerals. The quality of our diet is falling, and there is evidence to link this with increasing:

1  obesity
2  diabetes mellitus
3  hypertension
4  cardiovascular disease
5  appendicitis
6  dental decay.

---

## Vitamin content

The National Food Survey has shown that consumption of fresh fruit and vegetables has fallen over the last 30 years (Figure 10.1). The percentage reductions are shown in Table 10.1.

The foods mentioned are the main sources of vitamins A and C, which together with E and selenium form the body's defence against free radicals. Consumption of fresh fish and red meat, which also contain antioxidant substances –

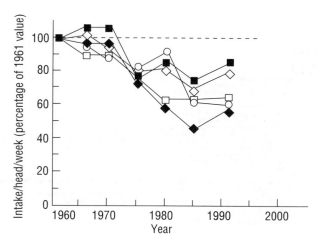

**Figure 10.1** Mean adult weekly intake of major foods, 1961–91, expressed as a percentage of 1961 levels.  □ Potatoes;  ◆ fresh vegetables;  ○ meat;  ◇ fish;  ■ fresh fruit. Source: Seaton A (1994) *Thorax*: 171–4. BMJ Publishing Group.

**Table 10.1** Percentage reductions in consumption of fresh food 1961–85

| Food | Reduction in consumption (%) |
| --- | --- |
| Fresh fruit | 26 |
| Green vegetables | 51 |
| Potatoes | 37 |

ubiquinones, selenium, zinc and copper – have also fallen. The fall-off of fish stocks has already been mentioned.

Not only have the quantities of fresh foods fallen, but also the quality of the food has declined. Schuphan[4] has argued, with evidence, that the EU drive to standardization and yield maximization has been to the detriment of the nutritional value of our food. Water is the only constituent of conventionally farmed produce to be increased when compared with organic produce. Figure 10.2 compares the mineral content of organic and commercial foods, showing an advantage on most counts for organic production. Given this fact, and the use of universally unpopular set-aside to reduce production, the failure of the EU and government to stimulate and encourage organic producers can only be described as bizarre.

# Minerals

Macrominerals such as calcium, phosphorus, magnesium, sodium, potassium and chloride ions are needed in quantity for general structural and functional purposes.

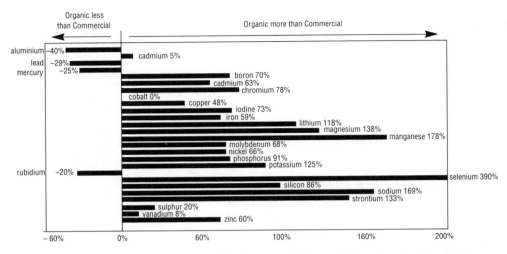

**Figure 10.2** Organic versus commercial foods. Source: Doctor's Data Inc., January 1993.

Micromineral or trace elements comprise a number of metals which are needed in tiny amounts to enable enzymes to function. They include iron, zinc, copper, manganese, iodine, chromium, boron, molybdenum, cobalt, sulphur and selenium. Other elements may yet be added to this list, including vanadium, nickel, tin and lithium. Figure 10.2 shows that levels for most of these micronutrients are higher in organic food than in the commercially produced equivalent,[5] and that the levels of three potential toxins were raised in commercial food, as against one (cadmium) in organic food.

This again argues in favour of organic food and, together with the gain in vitamins, the reduction in pesticide contamination, the reduction in soil erosion and the gain in rural employment levels associated with organic production, makes an overwhelming case for stimulating the production of organic food.

# Vegetarianism

The health of vegetarians in comparison with meat-eaters has been studied extensively, and overwhelmingly the result is that vegetarians on a properly balanced regimen are healthier in the following respects.

- They are less obese.
- They have lower blood pressure.
- They are less likely to suffer from coronary thrombosis.
- They suffer less from gastrointestinal cancer, especially colonic.[6]
- They have fewer gallstones.
- They suffer less constipation and diverticular disease.
- They have less trouble with diabetes and rheumatoid arthritis.

The vegetarian diet contains more fibre and antioxidant vitamins than the diet of meat-eaters, and levels of cadmium, mercury and lead are lower in the blood of vegetarians. There is, however, a risk of running low on calcium, zinc, selenium and the essential fatty acid docosahexanoic acid (DHA).

Ecologically, vegetables have the great advantage that the land area required to produce a given amount of protein is only one-twentieth of that required to produce the same amount of animal protein. In answer to this it is argued that animals are necessary to maintain the correct balance of the agricultural cycle.[7] However, the soil fertilization loop can be closed using clean recycled human sewage sludge, and in any case it is unlikely that the whole population will move to a vegetarian diet.

# Nutrition of pregnant mothers

Research in pregnant women[8] has shown that diet, especially around the time of conception, is related to the birth weight of the infant. It was found that diet became worse from social class I to V, and was worst of all for single mothers. In the worst diets, proteins, minerals and six B vitamins were lacking. Infants who were premature or suffered intrauterine growth retardation were born with deficits of two essential fatty acids (arachidonic acid and DHA) known to be required for brain development. It is also known that the health of the newborn infant is reflected in many aspects of health for the rest of the person's life.

The importance of this information can hardly be overstated. If there is the slightest chance that correction of deficiency of diet for nine months can prevent unhealthiness for the whole lifetime of the unborn child, society has a clear human and economic interest in making sure that deficiency is corrected. The payback on the investment, although not yet quantified, is bound to be over-whelming. There is clearly every reason to persuade prospective mothers to eat well, to the extent of providing supplements to those who cannot afford to.

# *Trans* fats

The debate about fats, cholesterol and heart disease rages on, generating more scientific heat than light. The idea that high saturated fat in our diets increases cholesterol in the blood, which is deposited in the lining of arteries, leading to coronary heart disease, is oversimplified.

It is modelled on people with familial hypercholesterolaemia (FH), who number about 1:500 of the population. They have a genetic deficiency of the lipoprotein receptors on their cell walls, meaning they are unable to take cholesterol out of the blood. Blood cholesterol rises and becomes deposited around tiny rips in the blood vessels, leading to coronary heart disease (CHD).

It was natural for doctors to extrapolate from the FH group to people at large, and to urge the lowering of saturated fats in the diet as a means of preventing coronary heart disease. More than 30 clinical trials have shown that this is not an effective strategy. Dr G V Mann[9] suggests that this is because the polyunsaturated fat diet used in these trials contains *trans* fats from hydrogenated oils, and that *trans* fats block cell lipoprotein receptors, creating artificially the conditions faced by people with FH.

In 1912, food technologists discovered how to hydrogenate polyunsaturated oils, turning them into fats. In the course of hydrogenation, 5–75% of the fatty acids are turned into *trans* fatty acids (TFAs). This refers to the configuration of the molecule; fats in mammalian tissues are normally in the *cis* configuration, with their side branches pointing in the opposite direction to those of the *trans* fats.

The increase in CHD began to be noticed in about 1920, and continued until the present day. The increase in CHD diagnoses was due in part to the advent of the electrocardiograph (ECG), and the condition certainly existed before 1920. However, the concentration of TFA in fat cells has been shown to be proportional to deaths from CHD.[10] The hypothesis explains national, age and sex differences in CHD, as well as the increase in insulin resistance seen in this century, and some other observations. Some recent work does not confirm the hypothesis, but the debate continues. It is probable that the outcome will be a recommendation for reduction in all fats of all kinds except fats derived from wild fish and the olive.

# Sugar

Davies and Stewart[1] provide evidence that sugar consumption is associated with the following problems:

1 obesity
2 cardiovascular disease (hypertension, raised blood fats, increased platelet stickiness, atherosclerosis)
3 diabetes mellitus (adult type)
4 gastrointestinal disease (indigestion, inflammatory bowel disease, diverticular disease, irritable bowel syndrome, gallstones)
5 kidney stones and failure
6 increased susceptibility to infection
7 reactive hypoglycaemia
8 depression and anxiety, childhood hyperactivity
9 seborrhoeic dermatitis, acne, dandruff, eczema.

By no means all of these connections are accepted as causal by the community of medical scientists, and it is not claimed that sugar is solely responsible in all individuals, but each association is backed by evidence.

In addition, sugar may lie behind the poor appetites of the nation's children. Many parents, doctors, dietitians and health visitors have found from practical experience that children who 'won't eat a thing that is put in front of them' recover their normal appetites when their supply of sugar and confectionery is curtailed.

In view of the multiplicity of conditions associated with excess sugar consumption, it would be reasonable and precautionary to take action to reduce the nation's intake of sugar. Indeed, the evidence to the 1983 NACNE report was so strong that a reduction of 50% in our sugar consumption was recommended.[11]

There is therefore a case to be made for government action in the form of disincentive taxes on sugar, hypothecated to medical research and to paying the bill for that proportion of dentistry that is judged to be due to sugar consumption.

# ADDITIVES

Food additives range from harmless adulterants such as water that are merely added in order to defraud consumers of their money, to dyes, which can make the lives of a minority of children and their families an absolute misery. Space does not allow for a detailed review of the hundreds of agents, but only a consideration of the assessment of the health risk and recommendations for government action.

## Adulterants

Adulterants have been added to food ever since the first innkeeper had the bright idea of increasing profits by watering his beer. Detailed legislation early in the twentieth century stopped most forms of adulteration, but it is still practised in the form of water added to processed meats to increase their weight. Often, polyphosphates are added, ostensibly to improve texture, but with a welcome (to the seller) side-effect that water can be sold at a premium. The London Food Commission estimates that, of £100 million fish fingers sold, £6 million will be added water.[12]

## Preservatives

Preservatives are added to food to stop it 'going off', as the name suggests. Without them, the food might become infected with micro-organisms. Preservative-free sausages will survive only one or two days in the fridge; with preservatives, four or five. There is therefore a rationale for the use of preservatives, and also for antioxidants, which prevent fats from tasting rancid. In fact, some antioxidants are natural vitamins, but doubts have been raised about the safety of other antioxidants.

## Cosmetics

Preservatives and antioxidants account for only 56 food additives. The rest – emulsifiers, stabilizers, colourings, flavours, flavour enhancers, sweeteners, texture modifiers, sequestrants and processing aids – add up to a total of at least 3740 different substances. None of these are strictly necessary for the nation's nutrition. True, without them some processed foods would not be marketable, since they would separate into their constituent parts, but this would not affect the nation's health: since most of them are sweet 'puddings' the result might be a healthy change towards fresh fruit.

In the case of at least one sweetener, aspartame, there is much doubt over the quality of the research that allowed it to come on to the market. The American Food and Drug Authority shared these anxieties in 1977, but did not pursue them. DKP, a breakdown product of aspartame, is thought to be toxic if taken in quantity, day after day, which is the case with some people.

If cosmetic additives are not necessary, is there evidence that they are harmful? The answer is clearly 'yes, some additives are harmful to some individuals'.

The debate on the effects of food additives on health is voluminous, with major contradictions between evidence provided by sceptics and that provided by believers. Sceptics are forced to admit that reactions to foods can occur, but they claim that this is very rare, and that most cases of 'food allergy' are mistaken. They rightly warn of the dangers that may result from following excessively and unnecessarily restrictive diets.

Physicians who practise environmental medicine argue that intolerance of additives is fairly common, and that effective avoidance diets, if checked by professionals, can be equal to or excel the nutrition of an open diet, although they are somewhat inconvenient.

The key question is whether additives, especially colourings and preservatives derived from coal tar, contribute to hyperactivity in childhood. Dr Joseph Egger, working at the Great Ormond Street Hospitals, has provided a definitive and positive answer to this question.[13] He selected 76 overactive children and put them on an 'oligoantigenic' (or 'few foods') diet. This is a diet which has empirically been found to be most unlikely to provoke reactions in any food-intolerant people. The children followed this diet for six weeks. Sixty-two (82%) improved, and the behaviour of 21 (28%) became normal. Other symptoms, such as headache, abdominal pain and fits, also improved. Next, the children were 'challenged' with foods that were thought to be provoking them. The challenge was a double-blind crossover placebo-controlled trial in which neither the child nor the clinician knew what the child was receiving. Twenty-eight of them (37% of the original sample) became worse when active food materials were given. Forty-eight different foods were incriminated. Artificial colourings and preservatives were the commonest provoking substances, but no child was sensitive to these alone.

Research in Australia[14] on 200 hyperactive children removed synthetic colouring from their diet. The parents of 150 claimed that they improved on this regimen. Fifty-four of the children were given either placebo or colouring, and 24 of these reacted to colouring with irritability, restlessness or sleeping difficulty. This would suggest that colouring is implicated in at least 25% of hyperactive children – a conservative estimate, since preservatives and other foods were implicated in Egger's study, and he found that partial elimination of provoking substances was less than partially effective.

The incidence of hyperactivity appears to be rising. A few years ago, a survey in the Isle of Wight found an incidence of 1:10 000 (0.01%) children. Currently hyperactivity (as attention deficit/hyperactivity disorder, ADHD) afflicts 3–4% of children in the UK. The figure in the USA is 10%. Some of this discrepancy may be due to differences in diagnostic categories, but since as a general rule the USA leads the world in allergies it may be that there is a genuine increase in incidence also.

One remarkable feature of the treatment of ADHD patients is that, despite the evidence that food exclusion is effective, ritalin, a stimulant related to the amphetamines, is given as a first-line treatment to children who have not been formally assessed for food intolerance. The drug is effective as long as the child takes it, but the condition recurs on stopping, and we have no knowledge of the long-term side-effects of the drug. In adults, long-term consumption of stimulants can lead to paranoid psychosis.

In 1989 there were 11.5 million children under the age of 16 in the UK. If 3% are hyperactive, this gives a figure of 345 000. If 25% (86 250) of these could be improved by elimination of colourants, a rough estimate for the cost of each case can be derived:

| | | |
|---|---|---|
| Three GP consultations @ £9.43 each | = | £28.29 |
| Six psychiatric outpatient consultations @ £48 each | = | £288.00 |
| Two social work visits @ £10 each | = | £20.00 |
| Total per case | = | £336.29 |
| × 86 250 cases | = | £29 005 012 |

An annual cost can be derived if it is assumed that each child is in therapy for four years out of 16:

$$£29\ 005\ 012/4 = £7\ 251\ 253 \text{ per year}$$

However, this would be a gross underestimate, since the stress caused by the child on the family will undoubtedly generate more demands on the NHS. A proportion of the children will be sent to special residential schools, with significant costs. Beyond the NHS, a proportion will go on to incur significant amounts of police, court and prison service time.

It must be remembered that even if intolerance to colouring is recognized – and in the vast majority of cases it is not – bonding between mother and child in the vital early years may have been adversely affected, causing continuing psychological problems despite having identified the biochemical problem.

It is not claimed that food intolerance is the sole cause of childhood overactivity, but this evidence certainly shows that it is a significant factor, and given the lack of alternative safe and effective treatments the only remaining puzzle is why more public money is not put into research along these lines.

## Recommendations

That colourings and preservatives found to cause reactions in more than 0.1% of the population should be banned outright and that the status of coal tar preservatives and all other food additives be thoroughly reviewed.

The full costs of treatment of 25% of hyperactive children, and the cost of further research into the relation between hyperactivity and food colourings and preservatives, should be met out of a levy placed on manufacturers of food dyes.

# Pesticides[15]

The term pesticide includes insecticides, herbicides, fungicides, molluscicides, growth regulators and seed dressings. They are used in agriculture, horticulture, forestry, fish farming, parks, gardens, playing fields, in fumigation and wood preserving, industrial pest control, flykillers, wallpaper pastes, tile grout, paint, masonry treatment, carpets and in medical preparations. In the production of non-organic food they are used as seed dressings during the growth phase (some products may receive as many as 30 applications) and during storage, so that almost the entire population is consuming minute (and sometimes not so minute) quantities of them as residues on a regular basis. They are hard things to avoid. The US Environmental Protection Agency estimates that 7% of all pesticides produced are used in the home and garden.

There are at least 600 pesticides which are presented in 45 000 different combinations. At least 37 have been judged to be safe by the US Environmental Protection Agency, which leaves 563 with a safety question mark hanging over their heads.

## Studying the effects on human health

Our knowledge of the effects of pesticides is inversely proportional to the number of people affected by them.

A very few cases occur of outright poisoning ('acute high-dose toxicity'): there is no doubt about the cause of the illness, the illness can be studied in detail and the effects are recorded in the toxicological textbooks.

More people are exposed to medium doses of pesticides during manufacture and application. The health of these groups of workers can be studied, and conclusions can be drawn, although with the familiar controversy as to when an association can be upgraded to a causal relationship. Manufacturing studies may involve only one pesticide, whereas applicator studies (of farmworkers, groundsmen, etc.) may involve exposure to a multiplicity of agents. The latter case may theoretically be more dangerous if synergy takes place, but the science needed to ascribe causality becomes more difficult. Nevertheless, most of what we know about medium-dose toxicity comes from occupational studies. The weakness of these studies is that of the 'healthy worker effect' – by definition, none of the study group are children, and few are pregnant or ill. Therefore, they tell us nothing about the effect of pesticides on these vulnerable groups.

The third group of exposed people is just about everyone on the planet, with the relative exception of one group. As shown above, we are all exposed to pesticides in what we hope are very low doses. In theory, the doses are so low that they do not affect us. The theory is weakened by considering the number of agents involved, the possibility of synergy and the fact that each of them is designed to act as a poison on living systems, with some being specifically designed to poison nerve transmission.

The theory that long-term, low-dose toxicity is not a problem has never been put to the test. It should and must be tested. Dr David Coggan, one of the UK's leading epidemiologists, has observed that if everyone smoked we would never have discovered that smoking is bad for us. To test the routine exposure that we all face through our food, we need a group who are not exposed in this way. Organic farmers and their families are the nearest approximation we have to this ideal group. Some organic (and this term should be taken to include permaculture and biodynamic practitioners also) farmers scrupulously avoid any food that is not organic: others are more easygoing in their habits. A study should be designed of the health of organic farmers, comparing them with a matched group of conventional farmers and, if possible, another group of outdoor workers – rangers, gamekeepers, countryside managers – who do not use pesticides. The comparison between farmers would show up any health variations owing to routine use of pesticides, which is an above average dose. Comparison between farmers' families would show up any differences that are ascribable to effects of the low doses given by, for instance, laundering pesticide-impregnated clothes: and the variation within the organic group between lifelong organic farmers and recent converts would tend to show up any subtle effects.

This research should be funded, on an arm's-length basis, by the pesticide industry, in accordance with the polluter pays principle.

## Known effects on health

Pesticides are among the pollutants that are described as xeno-oestrogens – foreign substances that have oestrogenic (feminizing) effects in the human body.[16] This subject will be considered on page 227.

Fourteen studies, mainly in the USA, of workers who use pesticides have thrown up relationships with some cancers. Table 10.2 shows the composited results.

**Table 10.2** Cancers associated with pesticide use (figure shows number of papers in which the association is found)

| | |
|---|---|
| Leukaemia | 8 |
| Multiple myeloma | 8 |
| Hodgkin's lymphoma | 1 |
| Non-Hodgkin's lymphoma | 8 |
| Lymphosarcoma | 2 |
| Reticulum cell sarcoma | 1 |
| Prostatic | 4 |
| Ovarian | 1 |
| Cervical | 1 |
| Stomach | 2 |
| Melanoma | 1 |
| Brain | 1 |

Source: *Pesticides, Chemicals and Health*[17]

One approach to the problem is to take known cancer patients and assess their past exposure to pesticides, comparing their use with that of control subjects without cancer. Three studies[18,19,20] have found that children with brain cancer are more likely to have been exposed to pesticides than control children, and one has shown a link with acute lymphocytic leukaemia. Two other studies[21,22] have failed to find a link. This kind of research is limited by the ability of people to recall their use of pesticides in the past.

The association with neoplasms of the immune system shown in the first block of six diagnoses in Table 10.2 is striking. It is difficult to escape the conclusion that pesticides help to cause cancers of the immune system. If this is the case, it is most likely that they also cause other, less easily detected, inefficiencies in immune system functioning, which would be manifested in increases in the number of bacterial and viral infections suffered by the population, which would be reflected in increasing anti-infectious medication use. Crude figures bear this out, since between 1981 and 1991 the cost of infectious and parasitic diseases (excluding respiratory tuberculosis) rose by 15.5% at 1991 prices adjusted to the NHS pay and price index. This observation is consistent with the hypothesis that our immune systems are growing less competent.

Organophosphorus-induced delayed polyneuropathy (OPIDIP) is a form of nerve weakness that persists after the acute effects of moderate poisoning have worn off.[23] Allied to this effect on nerves is an observed effect on memory, mood and 'abstraction'.[24]

Immune dysfunction induced by pesticides, long suspected by clinical ecologists, is documented in animal studies, and in humans by observed reduced immune response in women associated with levels of aldicarb at 16.6 parts per billion in their drinking water.[25]

## The cost of pesticide use

A precise estimate of the impact of pesticide use on NHS spending is not possible until the comparison of organic and industrial farmers has been made, but a conservative estimate might be set at 1% of the cost of treating cancers and 1% of the cost of treating infections. At 1991 prices, this yields costs of £14 000 000 per year to the NHS.

An exhaustive analysis has been made of the indirect costs of pesticide use in the USA.[26] Costs were considered under the following headings:

- human health
- livestock losses
- control expenses (loss of natural predators and pesticide resistance)
- pollination losses
- honeybee losses
- crop and product losses
- fish, wildlife and micro-organism losses
- government expenses to reduce costs.

It was concluded that human health impact incurred the greatest cost. Poisonings and cancers, but not immune system, fertility and hormonal effects were counted. The best estimate of the total indirect cost was $8 billion per year for the USA. The authors stressed the incompleteness of the data and that the true estimate would be 'significantly greater' than the $8 billion that they quoted.

The balance sheet for pesticide use is therefore as follows:

|  | $ billion |
|---|---|
| Financial cost of pesticide use | (4) |
| Indirect costs of pesticide use | (8) |
| Benefits in terms of crops saved | 16 |
| Net benefit | 4 |

Since research is still proceeding on the true indirect costs, it may well be that at the end of the day there is no net benefit whatsoever from using pesticides. Meanwhile, while the pesticide industry enjoys the profits from their use, it is society and the taxpayer that pick up the tab for investigating and treating the indirect effects of their product. It would be just therefore to apply a levy to all pesticides, hypothecated to research into, and treatment of, the indirect effects of pesticide use.

In less developed countries, the health toll is much greater owing to indiscriminate use, poor working practices and use of older pesticides that have been banned in the developed world. A net benefit is therefore likely to be even more doubtful.

# Caffeine

Caffeine is present in coffee (about 80 mg per cup), tea (about 60 mg per cup), cola drinks (about 30 mg per cup) and in small amounts in chocolate. It is an effective stimulant drug with a wide variety of effects which have been studied in some detail and reviewed by Battig.[27] The chief agreed effects are as follows.

1  Caffeine contributes to raised blood pressure and its effects on blood pressure and stress-related hormone systems are additive with stress.
2  Coffee consumption appears to elevate cholesterol levels slightly.
3  Coffee consumption appears to increase the relative risk of coronary thrombosis by a factor of up to 2.7.
4  Psychological tests of performance suggest that caffeine improves vigilance, slows reaction times, slows discrimination of ambiguous stimuli and may reduce memory for words. When test subjects are put under stress, it is found that, as expected, both high and low stress lead to reduced performance, but that the effects of caffeine are different in introverts and extroverts (see below).
5  Endurance and performance test outputs may be increased, although results were inconsistent.
6  Interindividual differences, as between caffeine users and non-users, and between introverts and extroverts, affects the result of tests.
7  Caffeine definitely reduces night-time sleep and daytime sleepiness.
8  It opposes the sedating and performance-reducing effects of benzodiazepines.
9  It probably stimulates the pleasure centres, making it mildly habit-forming.
10  It has a definite withdrawal syndrome, characterized chiefly by somnolence, fatigue and headache.
11  It is clearly implicated in the causation of migraine, and contributes to some cases of reflux oesophagitis (heartburn).

These research findings confirm the anecdotal observations of individuals and physicians who have noticed that in some people anxiety/stress symptoms can be reduced or eliminated by excluding caffeine from the diet. The fact that caffeine opposes the tranquillizing drugs, and may in fact act on the same nerve receptors, is an important clue.

Further studies support the idea that caffeine may contribute to anxiety/stress states. Kynurenine, a neurotransmitter related to anxiety, was found in the plasma of volunteers after a large dose of caffeine.[28] In a survey of 293 Japanese medical students, caffeine consumption was significantly and positively related with anxiety symptoms in males.[29]

In a rural general practice population of 2000 patients, 20 patients with symptoms of anxiety, insomnia or headache were asked to exclude caffeine from their diet (unpublished data). Of the 18 who complied, nine stated that they were to some degree better as a result of stopping caffeine. These cases may be taken as some crude indication of the incidence of caffeine-related disorders. Nine patients over four years out of a population of 2000 gives an incidence of 100 cases per year per 100 000 or an incidence of 50 000 for the whole of the UK. The age range of patients who were asked to stop was from 20 to 80 years, with the majority between the ages of 40 and 60. If it is assumed that the duration of symptoms were the coffee drinking to continue was 20 years, the prevalence of these symptoms would be 1 million, or 2% of the population of the UK. Assuming that the symptoms caused by caffeine would increase the GP consultation rate by 50% in this group, and given that the per capita cost of general medical services is £145, the estimated extra cost would be £72.60 per person affected per year, or £72 600 000 per year.

This estimate is, of course, based on an extreme extrapolation, but this crude methodology is compensated for by the fact that it is an extremely conservative figure since the hypertensive and coronary mortality figures have been left out of the calculation. If further studies confirm this figure, even within an order of magnitude, there is a clear case for applying a 'polluter pays' levy to caffeine products, to be applied initially to further research in this field, and, if the balance of probabilities indicates that caffeine is responsible for NHS costs, for a commensurate sum to be levied to recompense the NHS.

## Caffeine, introverts and extroverts

Revelle *et al.*[30] found that, whereas extroverts did better on verbal performance tests when dosed up with caffeine, introverts did worse.

In their experiment, the verbal ability of 100 students who had not consumed caffeine for six hours previously was tested in three ways.

1   They had to solve all 60 problems, taking as much time as necessary.
2   They had to solve problems as fast as possible, and were given placebo.
3   They had to solve problems as fast as possible but given caffeine.

The results showed that caffeine decreased the accuracy in introverted people but increased accuracy in extroverted people. This is consistent with other observations in extroverts receiving stimulant drugs.

It is a matter of concern to society that the introverted 30% of the population may be underperforming as a result of the effects of caffeine.

# Food poisoning

The incidence of episodes of food poisoning has been growing steadily since the mid-1980s, with a doubling of numbers every four to five years. An estimate for 1992, based on the government's figures multiplied by factors to allow for under-reporting, suggests a total of over 661 000, with 206 deaths. It is likely that the cause is multifactorial, with likely factors being:

1   automated decapitation, plucking and evisceration of chickens, which increases cross-contamination
2   lifestyle changes (more eating out)
3   consumerism changes (prewrapped foods)

4   cook–chill food preparation processes
5   increased reporting of cases.

Certainly the mass slaughter of chickens at the height of the salmonella scare did not solve the problem, since there was only a minor lessening of infections afterwards.

This increase is placing extra costs on the NHS. Assuming that one-third of the total number is an irreducible minimum, and that the two-thirds represents the increase over the last decade, we can cost the 400 000 'new' cases. The methodology and percentages are modelled on an assessment of the economic impact of an outbreak of dysentery.[31]

Costs of 400 cases of food poisoning

|  | £000s |
|---|---|
| 20% have their stools tested @ £15 | 1200 |
| 50% see GP once @ £8.95 | 1790 |
| 10% get home visit from GP @ £17.17 | 716 |
| 50% get rehydration powder @ £7.17 | 1434 |
| 5% get ciprofloxacin @ £7.50 | 150 |
| 10% receive four days' hospital treatment @ £138/day | 22 080 |
| 10% attend A&E @ £42 | 1680 |
| 5% get ambulance @ £106 | 2120 |
| Total | £31 190 |

This £31 million per year is an increased burden to the NHS which has been increasing over the last decade.

# Bovine spongiform encephalopathy

Bovine spongiform encephalopathy (BSE) or 'mad cow disease' is a condition marked by destruction of nerve cells accompanied by the production of two abnormal proteins, PrP and SAF.[32] It is new to cows, but has been known for many years as a disease of sheep called scrapie. It is clearly an infective disease, but the infective agent has not been identified. The existence of the infective agent is demonstrated when brain tissue from a suspect animal is injected into a mouse. It spread initially to cows through feeding them with dead sheep infected with scrapie. A total of 75 000 cows have been diagnosed with BSE, 90% of them dairy cows. Beef cattle do not live long enough to manifest the disease. Manifestly diseased animals are not allowed to be slaughtered for meat, but it is probable that infected carcasses do get through, either as a result of unscrupulous practices in the slaughterhouse, or because infected animals who are not yet showing signs of the disease are slaughtered and eaten. Brains and other infected tissues are removed, but the act of removal with circular saws inevitably deposits a spray of brain tissue on meat destined for the table.

Before March 1996 nobody knew for certain whether or not humans would be infected by consuming contaminated carcasses. The precautionary approach would have assumed that human infection was possible, until good evidence was found that proved otherwise. The government and its appointed scientific bodies chose not to use the precautionary approach. They pointed to the fact that there is no evidence that people have caught Creutzfeld-Jacob disease (CJD), the human equivalent of BSE, in areas where the sheep disease scrapie is rife. On this fact they founded their belief that there was no risk to the public from eating BSE infected meat. Only after a two-year delay did they bring in measures designed to exclude offal and central nervous system tissues from the human food chain.

Soon the BSE agent showed up in cats and zoo animals: evidence that it is capable of changing its characteristics and moving from species to species. This undermines the no-risk hypothesis and should have caused a switch to the precautionary approach. Instead, scientists who differed from the official line were themselves undermined. One scientist, Dr H K Narang, a Public Health Laboratory scientist in Newcastle, published work to show that the BSE agent, contrary to received thinking, did have DNA in its structure.[33] Moreover, he devised a urine test that promised to show quickly and easily which animals were infected. It is more than a little surprising that Narang's work was not followed up. Instead, his research funding dried up. Again, government policy had turned its back on the scientific approach based on new research in favour of the scholastic approach: 'the book says there is no risk, therefore there is no risk.'

Scientists of the precautionary school predicted that if BSE could lead to CJD, the earliest signs of an increase would be evident in 1996. In November 1995, cases of CJD were found in British teenagers,[34] whereas it is normally a disease of older people. This was not a good sign for the scholastic, no-risk theory. The death blow to the official line came in March 1996 when ten cases of a new, distinct strain of CJD were reported in humans. Instead of apologizing to the victims of their error, government spindoctors are at the time of writing conveying the impression that beef is now safe as cases of BSE are now falling to pre-1988 levels.

In the words of Sir Richard Southwood, chair of the government's working party on BSE, if CJD can be contracted by eating diseased beef 'the implications would be extremely serious'. In effect, the British beef-eating public are the subject of an experiment of uncertain outcome. The decision makers have gambled the mental health of the nation against the financial health of the British beef industry. It is now clear that the gamble has not paid off. The best outcome would be that government learns once and for all to take the precautionary approach in matters of this kind.

In a few years, we will have a clear idea of the cost of this failure to use a scientific and precautionary approach.

Due to the uncertainty of the outcome, no health costs can yet be ascribed to the BSE question.

## Cooking with microwaves

One study[35] showed that cooking with microwaves changed an amino acid, proline, from its natural L form to an unnatural D form. D-Proline has some toxic characteristics. The study was criticized on the grounds that the experimental substance (baby milk) was severely overcooked, and a subsequent study[36] could not replicate the findings. However, the second study used not food but solutions of the amino acid. Very little other work has been carried out on the effects of microwaves on food.

> ### Recommendation
>
> In view of the wide use of this kind of cooking, more research should be carried out into the effects of microwave cooking, funded on an arm's-length basis by a levy on the microwave cooker industry.

# DRUGS

A drug in the present context is any substance that alters the state of consciousness of a well human. The word 'well' is inserted (although it may be argued that a person who takes drugs is by definition not well) since sugar or other food can affect the state of consciousness of a person in diabetic pre-coma.

Addiction is the condition whereby an agent that affects behaviour creates its own need. This may be physical, withdrawal of the agent causing bodily or mental discomfort, or psychological, in which the use of the agent becomes an ingrained habit. Drugs are not the only agents of addiction: gambling, television, video gaming and even reading may equally create their own mental dependencies which isolate the addict from taking part creatively in the real world.

## Classification

Drugs may be broadly classified as stimulants, hallucinogens, tranquillizers, solvents and opiates.

1 Stimulants
   - tea
   - coffee
   - cocaine, crack cocaine
   - amphetamines

- MDMA (ecstasy)
- nicotine

2  Hallucinogens
- LSD
- mescaline
- (cannabis)

3  Tranquillizers
- benzodiazepines (Valium, Librium, nitrazepam, etc.)

4  Solvents (these operate by preventing nerve transmission by disrupting the fats lining the nerve cells)
- glue
- alcohol

5  Opiates (these constitute the class A drugs).

This classification is not absolutely watertight, for instance the solvent alcohol is thought to act by forming an opiate-like substance in the brain, whereas cannabis and nicotine possess both stimulant and tranquillizing properties.

## Alcohol

The social costs of alcohol misuse is £2.46 billion per year, to the NHS of £149 350 000 per year and the minuscule research budget of £800 000. Against these costs must be set the alcohol tax revenue, which yielded £8 961 900 000 in 1992–93, so that, unlike the motorist, it cannot be said that the drinker is under-taxed. The popularity (with the Treasury that is) of taxes on addictive substances such as alcohol and tobacco is that their addictive nature means that the tax does not erode its own base. On the other hand, this does not explain the undertaxation of motoring, which is also addictive.

In the UK alcohol consumption progressively increased from 4.4 litres of pure alcohol per capita per year in the 1960s to a peak in 1988–90 of 7.7 litres per capita per year, since when there has been a slight fall to 7.4 litres per capita in 1993.

As with tobacco, the issue of restriction of alcohol advertising has been suggested as a means of prevention of excessive drinking. It cannot be denied that the intrinsic purpose of advertising is to create a good image of, and good feeling about, a specific named drink in a proportion of any exposed population. In doing so, the same image and feeling suffuses alcohol itself. Of especial concern is the fact that beer advertisements are respectively second, third and fourth favourites with children aged 11–12, 9–10 and 6–8. There is a very clear case to be made for an outright ban on the advertising of alcohol in cinemas showing under-18 children's films and on TV before the 9 p.m. watershed.

As well as this measure, Alcohol Concern[a] is pressing for:

- the inclusion of health/safer drinking messages on TV advertisements
- a 10% levy on all alcohol advertising and sponsorship expenditure. This already happens in France. This would yield about £30 million to fund alcoholism prevention and education programmes.

To this might be added the requirement that all drinks labels should contain a small flash carrying one bit of information such as the sensible drinking limit or the effects of and penalty for drinking and driving.

Sponsorship of sporting events is worth about £180 million per year, and drinks companies supply about 10% of this. The association between alcohol and motor racing is clearly inappropriate, as is sponsorship of football, since alcohol is a factor in hooliganism that is the sport's greatest threat. Again, Alcohol Concern's objectives in this area are sensible and realistic.

Alcohol consumption is illustrated disproportionately frequently and positively in popular TV drama. The way to offset this bias would be a 'co-operative consultation' approach between broadcasters and alcohol educators. The aim would be to reduce inaccuracies, to halt the tendency to overglamorize drinking and to portray excess drinking in a way that shows the real consequences of that behaviour.

In conclusion, alcohol, despite being heavily taxed, still costs the nation dearly in health and social terms. Education that is more closely integrated with the process of alcohol promotion rather than leaflet campaigns carried out in a vacuum offers the best way forward.

# Class A (addictive) drugs

Addiction to hard drugs has been increasing steadily over recent years. Table 10.3 displays the trend for registered drug addicts – mainly for opiates.

The figures are for registered (notified) addicts. Many more do not register, and their numbers can be estimated from Home Office tables,[37] which show the (addictive) drug-related deaths for the UK. The ratio of all deaths to those of previously notified addicts is a fairly constant ratio of about 4:1 (range 3.4–4.4, average

**Table 10.3** Number of registered drug addicts in the UK

| Year | All addicts notified | Increase (%) |
|------|---------------------|--------------|
| 1990 | 17 755 | |
| 1991 | 20 820 | 14.7 |
| 1992 | 24 703 | 15.7 |
| 1993 | 27 976 | 11.6 |

[a] Alcohol Concern, Waterbridge House, 32–36 Lomand Street, London SE1 OEE.

3.9 for the years 1990, 1991 and 1992). The ratio for deaths involving class A drugs shoots up to 1:216.5 for 1991 suicide rates, and is high for suicide and undetermined deaths in all years, which suggests that people in the social circle of addicts may use their drugs to commit suicide.

## Costs

Prescription costs per addict are between £600 and £1200, and salary and office costs for a repeat prescribing and counselling clinic might come to £816 per client – making a total of between £1416 and £2016. For 27 296 cases the annual cost to the NHS is between £38 651 136 and £55 028 736. Since the numbers are growing by more than 10% per year, the drain on NHS resources is increasing to the tune of £46 million per year.

This is a conservative figure, since it does not include the extra cost of increased demand due to increased illness or the disproportionate consumption of GPs' time haggling for scripts.

In fact, the resources given to local drug problem teams are inadequate, and certainly not growing at a sufficient rate to keep pace with the demand, so the load falls back on to the GP, who suffers further stress and further losses in general efficiency.

The cost to society is even greater. If we take it that the number of unnotified addicts is 3 × 27 296 = 81 888 and assume that in their wild (unnotified) state they cost society three times what they would cost the NHS in prescribing and counselling, the cost is between:

$$81\ 888 \times £1416 \times 3 = £347\ 860\ 200 \text{ and}$$
$$81\ 888 \times £2016 \times 3 = £495\ 258\ 600 \text{ per year.}$$

The extra cost comes from increased theft and muggings carried out by addicts to pay for their supplies. Thefts cause emotional distress, insurance payouts and increased premiums, police, court and prison costs: muggings cause injury, severe emotional trauma, time off work, disability payments and criminal injury compensation payments.

From this it is clear that it is nine times more efficient to provide adequate resources for local drug problem teams than it is merely to deny that there is a problem or to give vent to ineffective punitive fulminations.

## Prevention

Availability of hard drugs is the main factor in the creation of drug addiction. Doctors and vets are the professional groups who are at most risk of becoming addicts not because they are inherently more depraved or stressed than lawyers, politicians and journalists, but because the drugs are available to them. Society must therefore attempt to stop drugs class A drugs coming on to the market. The attempt to do so by police and customs action has not succeeded.

An imaginative suggestion that has been put forward to stem the supply of opiate drugs at source is that government should buy the opium and cocaine crops from the hill farmers at a better price than is paid by the drug barons. This has been rejected by officials, but without good reason.

# Cannabis

There is evidence that increased cannabis use is associated with and may be caused by unemployment, although the evidence for alcohol consumption and unemployment is confused.

Cannabis is neither a hard drug nor an innocuous one. The side-effects of cannabis are:

1   criminalization of the user
2   association with addictive drugs, especially nicotine
3   inhalation as smoke
4   memory loss
5   'amotivation syndrome'
6   transient paranoia.

Serious although these effects are, it must be said that all drugs, licit or illicit, have side-effects, and in comparison with nicotine or alcohol the damage done by cannabis is minimal. Users would point out in particular that the effect of cannabis is to create an atmosphere of peaceable relaxation in which the enjoyment of conversation and music is the predominant feature.

Multiple sclerosis sufferers and those with a particularly severe form of glaucoma complain with great justification of the injustice of the present law which deprives them of access to a drug that is uniquely effective in controlling the effects of their illness.

## Criminalization

The greatest immediate risk to people who use cannabis is that they automatically become outlaws, with all that this implies for their integration into society. The question of the underclass is raised on page 112. To a large extent, cannabis is the preferred drug of the underclass, especially the black youth and 'traveller' groups. The present law is simply exacerbating the problem of social alienation.

On top of these incalculable social costs, there are very real costs of police, court and prison incurred in dealing with cannabis users who have the misfortune to be found out. Surprisingly, no government department admits to holding statistics on the cost of investigating, prosecuting and incarcerating cannabis users. The topic clearly needs to be subjected to an exhaustive cost–benefit analysis.

A further drawback of criminalization is that it tends to drive hard and soft drugs together. The higher levels of the chain of supply are likely to handle both cannabis and heroin, which means that an otherwise law-abiding person who has acquired a taste for an occasional mental unwind may be only one or two removes from criminals who carry deadly ironware when they go shopping for their supplies. Although the law drives hard and soft drugs together, cannabis culture generally makes a clear distinction. For instance, in the film *Easy Rider*, which takes a sympathetic view of dealing in cannabis, there is a song with uncompromising views on the demerits of the pusher of heroin.

Another drawback of the criminal status of the user is that research – especially field studies of people in their natural habitat, as opposed to laboratory studies – is inhibited. The upward trend in lung cancer noted below may be due to cannabis, but research will have more than the usual difficulties in establishing a causal relationship if patients are afraid to be candid. Similarly, doctors taking medical histories are misinformed because of the law, since users will deny taking the drug for fear of being misperceived or even reported by an establishment figure.

One of the more bizarre arguments is that some people seek the excitement of the illegal and that, if cannabis were to be decriminalized, they would transfer to other illegal drugs. This is on a level with the supposition that the fox enjoys being hunted. The corollary of the proposal is that boiled sweets should be made illegal to deflect the attentions of these hypothetical forensic masochists on to a substance that is only slightly harmful to health.

## Association with drugs of addiction

Although the fear that it may 'lead on to hard drugs' has been one of the key arguments against cannabis, despite a huge amount of research, a significant causal progression from cannabis to heroin has not been established. Dopeheads and junkies appear to form two separate subgroups, although naturally there is a degree of overlap between groups, and the law, as shown above, tends to increase the area of overlap.

Much more serious is the charge that cannabis leads on to nicotine addiction. It is undeniable that many sensible but adventurous youths first experience nicotine in a joint, and that the majority of these will continue to take tobacco as the carrier for cannabis or in the form of commercial cigarettes. This is a drawback, but tobacco is not a necessary part of ingestion, and in any case a society that tolerates tobacco advertising is not in a position to criminalize other ways in which people may become addicted to nicotine.

## Inhalation

The lungs were designed as a membrane to allow the transfer of oxygen inwards and carbon dioxide outwards. They were not designed as an ingestion route, and certainly not for the cocktail of tars produced by cigarettes and joints. There is evidence that synergy occurs between cannabis and tobacco smoke and a worrying upwards trend in lung cancer has been found in some sections of society which may be associated with cannabis use.

Cannabis can be eaten, which bypasses this problem, but this has its own draw-backs. Overdose of ingested cannabis causes an unpleasant weakness, with low blood pressure and weak pulse which, although not fatal, is very worrying. Education is needed to deal with this, but even here the law inhibits progress.

## Memory loss

Memory loss is a clear and common feature of heavy users. It is dose dependent so that heavy users suffer more than occasional users. Education therefore should be directed to the end of persuading users to give their brain cells regular and pro-longed breaks.

## 'Amotivation syndrome'

This is a term that has been used to describe a certain torpor and lack of drive dis-played by users which has been consistently observed. This is not to say that many highly motivated and successful individuals do not use cannabis as an effec-tive relaxant, so that 'hypomotivation' might be a more accurate term. It could be argued that, since unemployment is an integral and permanent part of the eco-nomic system (unless citizen's income is introduced), a happy acceptance of inac-tion is exactly what is needed, and that cannabis should be actively encouraged among the unemployed. It is possible that the prison service tolerates the drug for this reason.

The fact that the Legalise Cannabis Campaign is not more active and better sup-ported is probably a demonstration of the hypomotivation syndrome.

## Paranoia

It is well known in psychiatric circles that some susceptible individuals can respond to cannabis with brief psychotic episodes. Such persons should avoid the drug, and indeed they are usually only too happy to do so. (On the other hand, cannabis has been advocated in the past as a useful therapy to break up the rigid behaviour patterns of obsessive compulsive disease.) It may be also that all users display a low-grade paranoia, expressed in negative attitudes to society at large. Here again, the law in no way helps this problem, but rather institutionalizes it.

In summary, although cannabis, like all drugs, has its unwanted effects, there is no logic in its illegal status, and in fact this status serves to make things worse. It is probable that the underlying anxiety of society is that, if decriminalized, its use will become much more prevalent. This depends on three factors.

1   Most people who are curious about cannabis have already tried it; people who like to feel in control instinctively avoid it, so the scope for major increases in use is not great.
2   Education about its effects disseminated at the same time as decriminalization will deter many current non-users from taking it up and may even persuade some users to cut down or give up.

3   The alternative to illegality is not availability over the counter at the local tobacconist. Regulation, as with alcohol, is a possibility, and most users would probably be prepared to take a chance with registering as a user – the risk being that if a government of a more repressive nature came in their cover would be blown. Registration would enable prospective social and economic studies to clarify the exact impact of the drug on health: *in vivo* studies as it were instead of the *in vitro* studies hitherto carried out in the laboratory.

In the end, if smoking cannabis is a crime, the victim is the body and head of the perpetrator. If government considers that this is a proper area for legislation, it will have a busy time ahead protecting us from the many other self-damaging moral and spiritual imperfections that beset our times.

## Raves and the law

A nice piece of sequential logic decrees that raves should be legalized. Raves are dances attended by large numbers of young people, many of whom dance for long periods. A rare side-effect of the drug MDMA ('ecstasy'), taken often by some of the dancers, is fatal cardiac arrest. Dehydration brought on by continuous dancing contributes to these fatalities. To reduce these deaths, it is necessary to ensure that water is available free of charge to ravers. If the raves are illicit, the power to regulate the distribution of water is lost. Therefore raves should be licensed in the name of the sanctity of human life.

## CONCLUSION

In this brief tour of the things that we place in our internal environment, we have seen that we are casually tampering with a vastly complicated system, and despite much research, have only begun to understand the real effects of our actions. What is clear however is that certain diseases are on the increase, almost certainly as a result of our tamperings.

## REFERENCES

1   Davies S and Stewart A (1987) *Nutritional Medicine*. Pan, London.

2   West R (1994) *Obesity. OHE Paper 112*. OHE, London.

3   Seidell J C (1995) The Impact of Obesity on Health Status: some implications for health care costs. *Int J Obes*: **19(6)**; 513–16.

4    Schuphan W (1975) Yield maximization versus biological value. Problems in plant breeding and standardization. *Qual Plant Pl Fds Hum Nutr*: **XXIV**; 281–310.

5    Smith B L (1993) Organic foods *vs* supermarket foods: element levels. *J Appl Nutr*: **45**; 1.

6    Nair P and Mayberry J F (1994) Vegetarianism, dietary fibre and gastrointestinal disease. *Digest Dis*: **12**; 177–85.

7    Gussow J D (1994) Ecology and vegetarian considerations: does environmental responsibility demand the elimination of livestock? *Am J Clin Nutr*: **59(Suppl 5)**; 1110s–16s.

8    Wynn S W, Wynn A H, Doyle W *et al.* (1994) The association of maternal social class with maternal diet and the dimensions of babies in a population of London women. *Nutr Health*: **9**; 303–15.

9    Mann G V (1994) Metabolic consequences of dietary trans fatty acids. *Lancet*: **343**; 1268–71.

10   Thomsa L H (1975) Mortality from atherosclerotic disease and consumption of hydrogenated oils. *Br J Prevent Soc Med*: **29**; 82–90.

11   Health Education Council (1983) *Nutritional Guidelines for Health Education in Britain*. Health Education Council, London.

12   London Food Commission (1988) *Food Adulteration and How to Beat It*. Unwin, London.

13   Egger J, Graham P J, Carter C M *et al.* (1985) Controlled trial of oligoantigenic treatment in the hyperkinetic syndrome. *Lancet*: **1**; 540–5.

14   Rowe K S and Rowe K J (1994) Synthetic Food Colouring and Behaviour: a dose response effect in a double blind, placebo controlled, repeated measures study. *J Paediatr*: **125(5)**; 691–8.

15   Dinham B (1993) *The Pesticide Hazard. A Global Health and Environmental Audit*. Zed Books, London.

16   Raloff J (1993) Ecocancers: do environmental factors underlie a breast cancer epidemic? *Sci News*: **144**; 10–13.

17   Morgan D R (1992) *Pesticides, Chemicals and Health*. BMA Press, London.

18   Davis J R, Brownson R C, Garcia R *et al.* (1993) Family pesticide use and childhood brain cancer. *Arch Environ Contam Toxicol*: **24**; 87–92.

19   Gold E, Gordis L, Tonascia J *et al.* (1979) Risk factors for brain tumours in children. *Am J Epidemiol*: **109(3)**; 309–19.

20   Sinks T H (1985) N-Nitroso-compounds, pesticides, and parental exposures in the workplace as risk factors for childhood brain cancer: a case-control study. Dissertation. *Abstr Int*: **46(60)**; 1888–90.

21   Preston-Martin S, Yu M C, Beenton B *et al.* (1982) N-nitroso compounds and childhood brain cancer: a case-control study. *Cancer Res*: **45**; 5240–5.

22   Howe G R, Burch J D, Chiarelli A M *et al.* (1989) An explanatory case-control study of brain tumours in children. *Cancer Res*: **49**; 4349–52.

23   Lotti M (1984) The delayed polyneuropathy caused by some organophosphorus esters. In: C L Galli, L Manzo, P S Spencer (eds) *Recent Advances in Nervous System Toxicology*. Proceedings of the NATO Advanced Study Institute on Toxicology of the Nervous System. December 10–20. Belgirate, Italy. pp. 247–57.

24   Savage E P, Keefe T J, Mounce L W *et al.* (1988) Chronic neurological sequelae of acute organophosphorus pesticide poisoning. *Arch Environ Health*: **43**; 38–45.

25   Fiore M C, Anderson H A, Hong R *et al.* (1986) Chronic exposure to aldicarb contaminated groundwater and human immune function. *Environ Res*: **41**; 633–45.

26   Pimental D, Acquay H, Biltonen M *et al.* (1993) Assessment of environmental and economic impacts of pesticide use. In: *The Pesticide Question: Environment, Economics and Ethics*. Chapman & Hall, New York.

27   Battig K (1991) Coffee, cardiovascular and behavioral effects, current research trends. *Rev Environ Health*: **9**; 2.

28   Orlikov A and Ryzov I (1991) Caffeine-induced anxiety and increase of kynurenine concentration in plasma of healthy subjects: a pilot study. *Biol Psychiatry*: **29**; 1–6.

29   Mino Y, Yasuda N, Fujimura T *et al.* (1990) Caffeine consumption and anxiety and depressive symptomatology among medical students. *Arukoru Kenkyu-To Yakubutsu Ison*: 25; 486–96.

30   Revelle W, Amaral P, Turiff S (1976) Introversion – extroversion, time stress, and caffeine. Effect on verbal performance. *Science*: **192**; 149.

31   Creedon J and Murphy G (1993) Economic impact of dysentery. *Environ Health*: **June**; 176–8.

32   Lacey R (1994) *Health and the Environment*. Oxford University Press, Oxford.

33   Narang H K (1994) Evidence that homologous ss DNA is present in scrapie, Crentzfeld-Jacob disease and bovine spongiform encephalopathy. *Ann NY Acad Sci*: **754**; 314–26.

34   Bateman D, Hilton D, Lowe S *et al.* (1995) Sporadic CJD in an 18 year old in the UK. *Lancet*: **346**; 1155.

35   Lubec G, Wolf Chr, Bartosch S (1989) Amino acid isomerization and microwave exposure. *Lancet*: **9**; 1392–3.

36   Fritz P, Gehne L I, Zagon J *et al.* (1992) The question of amino acid isomerization in the microwave field. Results of a model study with standard solutions. (German.) *Zeitschrift für Ehrnarungswissenschaft*: **31**; 219–24.

37   Home Office (1994) *Home Office Statistical Bulletin. Issue 10/94*, London.

# 11
# Work in progress

It is certain that some diseases are increasing steadily, and alleged that environmental agents are causing other diseases to increase. This chapter tries to unravel the complexities of the debate.

## ASTHMA

Asthma causes 1700 deaths per year in the UK. Compared with 100 000 deaths per year from tobacco smoking and 4000–5000 from road accidents this is not a huge number, but it also causes uncounted disability, anxiety and misery. The economic cost to the UK of asthma has been calculated at about £1 billion per year:

| | | |
|---|---|---|
| Cost to NHS | = | £500m |
| Lost productivity | = | £350m |
| Social Security payments | = | £60m |
| Schooling | = | £1m |
| Total | = | £1bn |

These costs are rising rapidly. The cost of asthma medication alone rose from £305 million in 1992 to £381 million in 1994.

## Increasing prevalence

It is established that the prevalence of asthma has increased greatly in the twentieth century (Figure 11.1). For instance, a 141% increase in Australia has been recorded in the 27 years before 1991.[1] In Finland the percentage of military recruits with asthma has increased 20-fold since 1961.[2] Cases requiring inpatient treatment have risen 2.5-fold in 12 years. The biggest increases in the UK have occurred in the West Midlands and South West (Parliamentary answer, January 1994). One in ten of the population of Leicester is now diagnosed asthmatic. Despite improved treatments, several countries note an increase in asthma-related deaths.

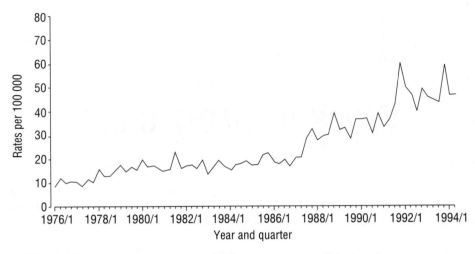

**Figure 11.1** Newly diagnosed episodes of asthma, average weekly rates, by quarter. Source: OPCS.

This increase cannot be explained solely by doctors becoming more aware of the possibility of asthma as a cause of their patients' symptoms – the so-called 'diagnostic shift'. There is a real increase in the disease, and since the blame cannot be placed on a change in our genetic make-up, the cause must originate in the environment. To determine the cause of this simple truth is not simple.

## Investigating the increase

The investigation of asthma itself is fraught with many complexities and difficulties, beginning with the lack of a 'gold standard' diagnostic test (such as an indisputable blood test) to establish that the condition is in fact present. Hospital records of admissions may show variable diagnoses in the same patient. One person may be given diagnoses of asthma or wheezy bronchitis on successive admissions to hospital. To make matters worse for researchers, there are confounding factors such as smoking, diet, occupation, geography and meteorology. Other difficulties are the poor standard of air quality (AQ) monitoring in the UK and the varied nature of the pollutants themselves ($O_3$, $SO_2$, $NO_X$, PM10, PM2.5) which have been studied individually and in pairs in the laboratory, but are experienced in multiple combination in real life. Synergy (one factor making the other worse) occurs between at least two agents[3] and there is a time delay of 24–48 hours between exposure to ozone and PM10 and their effects. All of these circumstances do not make for easy science. In an effort to tighten up on the criteria, the term 'bronchial hyper-reactivity' is sometimes used by researchers instead of asthma, since it is a specific and testable term.

There are two components to the increase in illness caused by asthma:

1 the increased number of people who suffer from asthma
2 the increase in the number of episodes of asthma suffered by asthma patients.

## The causes of the increase in new cases

It is highly unlikely that the increased prevalence of asthma (that is the increased number of people suffering from the condition) is due to any one single factor.[4] It is the result of a combination of several factors, of which the most likely candidates are:

- indoor air pollution
- outdoor air pollution
- diet
- occupation.

### Indoor air pollution

House dust mite is probably the most important factor in the generation of new cases of asthma. Some of the evidence for the allergenicity and increase in this unwanted lodger with whom we share our houses is set out on page 168. Increasing numbers of house dust mite explain why asthma has increased in parts of the world where the outside air is relatively pure, such as the Scottish highlands.[5] The distribution of increase in prevalence matches the geographical distribution of house dust mite fairly well.

Tobacco smoke appears to be implicated in the increase in allergy. Immunoglobulin E (IgE) concentrations are greater in the serum of smokers, and studies have shown that workers who smoke are at increased risk of developing allergies to inhaled allergens.[6] Mothers who smoke bear babies with diminished lung function and increased IgE. The increase in asthma in the West coincides with the increase in smoking in women of childbearing age.[7]

Other components of indoor air pollution may be implicated, including the use of perfumes. Many asthmatic patients complain that their chests become tight when they are exposed to the very strong synthetic perfumes in body deodorant sprays and domestic 'air fresheners'. Allergy to dog and cat fur and dandruff can cause asthma, but if sales of pet food are anything to go by ownership of pets has not increased enough to account for the increase in asthma.

### Outdoor air pollution[8]

Traffic pollution has in the past been dismissed as a possible cause of asthma by some authorities because pollution levels have been falling while asthma has been rising, and because the prevalence of asthma is increasing in countries and areas[5] where the air is relatively clean. The latter argument is compelling, but the 'falling pollution levels' argument is not so convincing, as the pollutants quoted are the old classics – sulphur dioxide and smoke. These pollutants are associated with chronic bronchitis rather than asthma, as is neatly demonstrated by the different pollution and disease levels in East and West Germany.[9,10] There are, however, a newer group of pollutants whose advent coincides with the increase in asthma – road traffic emissions, especially nitrogen oxides, ozone and diesel smoke.

Diesel smoke, like all smoke, consists of particles of carbon, but the particle size for diesel is unusually small – less than 10 microns in diameter ('PM10s'), and some are less than 2.5 microns ('PM2.5s'). This small particle size means that they can penetrate deep into the lungs, instead of being deposited in the nose or upper airways, which is the fate of larger particles. A possibility which is currently being researched is that diesel smoke particles may have specific properties that cause it to affect the electrical polarities of some molecules with which it comes into contact in a unique way.

Warren Spring Laboratory estimates that diesel smoke in the UK has doubled between 1970 and 1989 to a total of 182 000 tonnes per year. Petrol engines bring the total from road transport up to 198 000 tonnes per year.[11] Diesel engines are 100 times smokier than petrol. This increase undermines the argument that asthma has been rising while pollution has been falling, and leaves traffic-generated particles in contention as contributors to the increased prevalence of asthma.

In Japan there is a road that runs through a forest of Japanese red cedar. Many who live there are allergic to the pollen of the tree, but the incidence of allergy is three times greater in those who live close to the road than in those living deep in the forest.[12,13] This suggests that traffic pollution combined with natural antigens such as pollen is effective in switching on allergies. The study supports the view that traffic pollution may have something to do with the increase in cases – prevalence – of asthma, as well as exacerbations of established cases. However, the study has been criticized on the grounds that socioeconomic factors may have confounded the results.

Japanese scientists went on to study the effects of diesel smoke particles in laboratory animals. They found that diesel smoke together with pollen was 100 times as effective in raising levels of the allergen globulin IgE as pollen alone. Berciano et al.[14] confirmed that pollution levels in the environment corresponded to IgE levels in local children.

Other components of traffic pollution may also contribute to the production of allergies. Nitrogen dioxide in high doses (higher than found in town air) has been shown to interfere with tolerance induction, that is to make it more likely that an individual will become allergic to an antigen. As well as being found in the street, nitrogen dioxide is also produced in the kitchen from gas stoves. It is possible that this gas has been contributing to the increase in respiratory allergy, although it must be said that most effects have only been found at levels much higher than those found in the environment.

## Occupation

The Health and Safety Executive has found that chemicals encountered in industry can cause sensitization and asthma irrespective of the effects of smoking and allergies to pollen and house dust mite. The most common of these are isocyanates, flour dust, laboratory animal urine proteins, wood dust and solder flux. The Surveillance of Work and Occupational Respiratory Disease project believes that occupational sources are responsible for between 1500 and 2500 new cases of asthma each year.[15]

# The cause of increased episodes of asthma

## Outdoor air pollution

People who have been diagnosed as having asthma may continue to be well for months or years owing to a combination of avoidance of challenging situations and good medication. Alternatively, they may suffer repeated episodes of difficulty in breathing. Whatever its role in causing new cases of asthma, it is pretty clear that outdoor air pollution is a substantial contributor to the problem of exacerbations of established asthma.

Schwartz and Dockery[16] found that in several US cities over a ten-year period daily mortality rates showed a positive correlation with the level of PM10s in the air the previous day. The study took careful account of potential confounding factors such as temperature and humidity. The findings were very consistent between cities with a rise in the overall death rate of 6–7% for every 100 $\mu g/m^3$ increase in total suspended particulates (TSPs). The effect was greater in the elderly and for those with cardiorespiratory diseases. No threshold was seen for the effect, which was still evident below ambient air quality guidelines, and three-to-five-day moving average pollutant levels were mostly associated with mortality.

Schwartz undertook a further study in Seattle, which showed an association between low levels of the previous day's PM10s and emergency room (i.e. accident and emergency) visits for young adults.[17]

Respiratory infections (which can in turn cause exacerbations of asthma) also rise in proportion to air pollution. Other work[18] shows that respiratory infections in children are related to air pollution. Dr Ardern, a community physician in Manchester, found that the major source of air pollution for Manchester Airport was private road traffic, and that pollution so generated was reflected in hospital admission rates. She has also compared asthma emergency admissions (ruling out wheezing and bronchitis) with $NO_2$ levels, choosing this pollutant because it was easy to measure. The correlation was 8.8 – a significant association.[19]

There is therefore good evidence that, whatever its contribution to the increased prevalence of asthma, traffic-derived pollution certainly contributes in a major way to the observed increase in episodes of asthmatic attack.

Our understanding of the ways in which this happens has increased as we understand more about the effects of free radicals (p. 158).

## Diet

Diet-increased salt intake has been associated in studies with adult mortality due to asthma. Salt has also been related to airway hyper-responsiveness, and lowered salt intake has been associated with lowered airway hyper-responsiveness. Salt is also implicated in high blood pressure.

---

### Recommendation

That a tax should be placed on salt, hypothecated to the NHS, equivalent to the best estimates of the amount of NHS spending commitment caused by salt intake. A maximum allowable salt level in tinned and other prepared foods should be set.

---

Antioxidant vitamins (A, C and E) are lacking in our diets (p. 192). Seaton[20] and co-workers have argued that this is important for asthma on the following grounds.

1  Inflammation associated with T-lymphocytosis is a feature of the asthmatic airway.
2  Inflammation may decrease tolerance and increase the likelihood of allergic sensitization.
3  Free radicals are generated in inflamed tissue.
4  The lung's free radical scavenging system depends on vitamins A, C and E, together with the minerals selenium, zinc and copper.

Relative lack of antioxidant vitamins combining with an increased free radical load from, among other things, air pollution will act together to increase airways inflammation which is one of the basic processes of asthma – another example of synergy.

Omega-6 fatty acids present in margarine spreads have also been blamed for the rise in asthma.[21] This constituent of sunflower oil is more proinflammatory and spasmogenic than other fatty acids.

Food intolerance and allergy may account for some of the cases seen. Australian researchers point out that apples, pears, carrots, potatoes, celery and nuts all carry proteins which are similar to birch pollen antigens. Clinical ecologists routinely treat asthma patients with food exclusion diets.

---

## Conclusion

Scientific consensus on the exact relationships of the many factors that are coming into play over the causation of asthma and exacerbations of established asthma is a long way off. Figure 11.2 shows the interplay of some of the factors implicated in asthma. Consensus will be easier to achieve if the quest for a single cause is dropped, and a multifactorial or 'system' solution is sought. There are still many questions that need to be answered by research, but government need not wait for the question of causation to be settled to the satisfaction of the academics: action to reduce the two main candidates, house dust mite as cause of increased

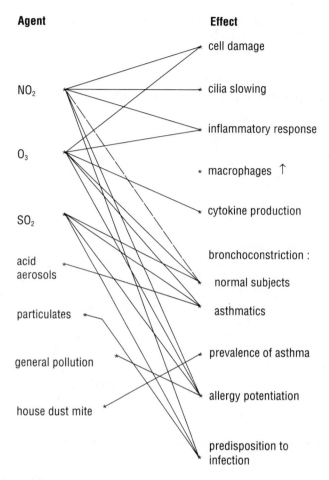

**Figure 11.2**  Interplay of factors in asthma.

prevalence and traffic-generated air pollution as cause of exacerbation, may reasonably be expected to:

1   reduce the discomfort of asthmatics
2   reduce NHS expenditure on asthma-relieving drugs
3   yield useful clues to the final question of causation itself.

Behind the scientific and political argument on air pollution lies the question of a value judgement relating to the contribution to the motor car to our quality of life. The misperception that the car contributes to the economic well-being of the country (the opposite is true) is still widely held even by educated people, and this affects the perception of what is to be done. On the other hand, action to reduce air pollution, even if it only produced a marginal improvement in asthma-related NHS costs, would significantly improve the quality of life for city dwellers, and this would in turn produce benefits to the NHS.

## FALLING SPERM COUNTS AND OTHER HORMONAL PROBLEMS

Recently there has been growing conviction among environmental scientists that we are facing a widespread problem with man-made chemicals that mimic the effects of female sex hormone, oestrogens.

The evidence is:

1   decreasing sperm quantity and quality in many studies
2   trebled rate of testicular cancer in 30 years
3   increasing incidence of undescended testicles in boys (doubled in 30 years) and feminization of the male fetus (hypospadias)
4   increasing incidence of prostatic cancer
5   increasing incidence of breast cancer (doubled in 30 years).

There is a model for this type of abnormality in medical experience with the drug diethylstillboestrone (DES), a synthetic oestrogen that produced the same kind of problems in the offspring of women who took it.

Reproductive effects have also been found in alligators, eagles, herons, frogs, polar bears, turtles and dolphins, showing how widespread the impact of man-made chemicals has become.

## Sperm counts

Several studies have shown that sperm counts have fallen significantly over the past 50 years. For instance, Dutch research[22] found that men who used carbaryl, benomyl and thiram to spray fruit took longer to make their wives pregnant. Twenty-eight per cent of those with high exposure and 8% of those with lower exposure were sufficiently worried to consult their doctors about this.

It is a relief to find a health index that is so clear-cut as the sperm count, but even with this there has been hot debate over the interpretation of results. Criticism has centred on the fact that counts will vary with the length of time since sperm was last ejaculated and the impossibility of cross-checking sperm records of 50 years ago on this point. However, the evidence is becoming stronger with each new finding, the vast majority of which points to a fall in quality and quantity of 'modern' sperm.

Having established that counts are indeed falling, the next question is: 'what is the reason for the fall?'. Sedentary lifestyle has been suggested, since in sitting the testes are kept in warm proximity to the body, whereas nature intended them to be cooled by breezes circulating beneath the kilt for optimum production. This warming may be a contributory factor, but does not account for the remarkable difference between sperm counts between organic and pesticide-using farmers which was found in the Dutch study.

# Xeno-oestrogens

This began a search for chemicals in the environment which had oestrogenic properties. So far, the following chemicals fit the bill:

- dioxins, furans, PCBs, PBBs, bisphenol A
- herbicides (2,4-D, 2,4, 5-T, atrazine), fungicides, BHCH (lindane, quellada), DDT, DDE, kelthane, heptachlor, kepane, methoxychlor
- cadmium, lead and mercury
- nonylphenol, a widespread chemical used as an antioxidant in plastics, and in detergents, paints, lubricating oils, toiletries – and as a contraceptive spermicide. About 20 000 tonnes are produced in the UK alone. It persists in the environment and concentrates in animal tissues.

One lesson to be learned from this episode is that in environmental chemistry the only thing that can be predicted is that unpredictable things happen. No one, looking at the above list of chemicals, could have predicted that they could affect our hormones. They might have been intensively studied for their carcinogenic potential, but that was of no help in predicting their endocrine (hormonal) effects. We have an inkling that some of them affect mammalian immune systems. What other unsuspected effects will come to light in the future?

## Dioxins

The term 'dioxin' is used as shorthand for polychlorinated dibenzodioxins, of which there are 75 types, and polychlorinated dibenzofurans, which number 135. It is easy to see why the shorthand form is used. Their pathogenic properties have not yet been exhaustively studied, but enough is known to regard them as highly toxic in very low doses. TCDD is one of the most potent carcinogens known to animal studies, yet it shows inter-species differences, with humans being a relatively resistant species. The same does not necessarily follow for all the other types of dioxins and furans.

They are widespread in the environment, and almost entirely man-made. Dioxins are present in bleached paper products, including disposable nappies, and as contaminants in the herbicides 2,4,5-T and PCP. Their main route of formation is through incomplete combustion of materials containing chlorine – especially PVC and PCBs. Traces of copper enhance its formation. To stop dioxins forming, it is necessary to hold exhaust gases at specified high temperatures for a specified length of time.

Most dioxins are bound to solid particles in smoke, and so can be captured in dust filter bags, providing the bags do not clog, stretch or break. This leaves the problem of what to do with the toxic accumulated ash, but at least the ash can be stored until new processes that can eliminate the dioxins completely are developed.

Monitoring and control of dioxins is problematical, as the chemical test for their presence is complex and expensive, and can only be carried out intermittently. It has been shown[23] that the cancer-producing potential of ash varies greatly over time, so that intermittent testing may miss past peaks and troughs in output.

The official list of dioxin sources in order of importance is as follows:

1   hospital waste incinerators
2   forest fires
3   industrial wood burning
4   diesel emissions
5   leaded fuel burning
6   residential wood burning
7   copper smelting
8   waste incinerators.

This list has been criticized on the grounds that it concentrates only on inhalation and omits consideration of the food chain as a source of dioxins. They accumulate as they pass up the food chain, so that top predators such as humans receive a concentrated dose. They are present in milk, both cow and human.

Dioxins have been shown to cause cancers and birth defects in animals. The developmental effects in mammals include decreased growth, structural malformations (that is birth defects, which occur at moderate and high doses), 'functional alterations' and prenatal mortality. The functional alterations are the most sensitive indicator of low-level toxicity, and include reproductive effects – lowered sperm count and abortions.

One important feature of dioxins is the fact that they are fat soluble, and therefore stored in body fat. During periods when fat is being absorbed, for example during weight loss diets and periods of illness, the dioxins will be released into the bloodstream.

In humans, the only effect that is generally accepted with certainty to result from dioxin exposure is chloracne, a painful eruptive skin condition. This was widespread around Seveso, the Italian region contaminated by a leak from a chemical plant. Birth defects were not seen as many mothers had preventive abortions. US servicemen contaminated by Agent Orange, a defoliant sprayed on the countryside in the Vietnam war, complained of reproductive effects, but failed to get a causal link officially accepted until 1996. It must be said that had the US war machine accepted responsibility it would have been faced with a huge compensation bill, and the perception remains that the true effects have been covered up.

Less certain than chloracne, but still under investigation, is the connection between dioxins and cancer, immunosuppression and reproductive toxicity in humans. Cancers of the stomach and sarcomas and lymphomas have been associated with dioxin exposure. This association has been challenged by Gough,[24] who compared levels of stomach cancer in herbicide workers and chemical plant workers. The latter had higher levels of exposure, but roughly the same level of stomach cancer. Gough deduced that the causal hypothesis would require the chemical plant workers to have higher levels. However, synergy between the dioxin contaminant and the herbicide itself cannot be ruled out, and so his argument does not necessarily prevail. Nevertheless, he has made the important point that measurements of dioxin in body fat, or at least the presence of chloracne as an indicator of exposure, is necessary before epidemiological inferences can be drawn about dioxin exposure.

Immunosuppression is a possible effect in humans. Because it is not such a definite clinical effect as cancer, being a grey area passing from increased susceptibility to coughs and colds to severe inability to fight off infections, it is not so easily studied.

In conclusion, much uncertainty still exists about the precise impact of dioxins on human health. They are so widespread that it is not easy to study them, since there is no 'clean' population to act as a control group.

## Pesticides

Pesticides are accepted to have oestrogenic properties.[25] The familiar DDT (dicophane), which is stored in body fats as DDE (dichlorodiphenyldichloroethylene), and polychlorinated phenols are examples of this group. Mortality from breast cancer in Israel declined after DDT and other pesticides ceased to appear in milk products.[26]

The mode of action of these xeno-oestrogens may be a disturbance of the ratio of oestrogenic to progesteronic effects in the body. Women with low levels of progesterone have been found to have a 5.4-fold increased risk breast cancer compared with those with higher levels of progesterone – and also a ten-fold increased risk of death from all malignant neoplasms.[27]

# DEPRESSION AND ANXIETY

There is a wealth of evidence to show that stress-related conditions – anxiety and depression – are increasing.

1   An OPCS survey indicates that one in seven people will suffer depression during their lifetime.[28]
2   There has been a 71% increase in suicide in young men in the UK over the last ten years.
3   Calls to the Samaritans have increased by 30% over the last ten years.

4   Hospital admission for children aged less than ten for psychiatric problems have increased by 50% over the last ten years.
5   There have been more hospital admissions for depression in the second than in the first half of the twentieth century.
6   'Grunge' pop song lyrics and letters to fan magazines, are filled with depressive content.

Paradoxically, this increase is not reflected in general practice consultations statistics for depression, which were 30% lower in men in 1991 when compared with rates for 1981, and 38% lower for women. In the face of the other evidence, it must be that people are not calling on the GP with depressive symptoms, but going to alternative therapists or none. Part of the solution may be a change in symptom presentation or diagnostic habits since, although both anxiety and depressive diagnoses have fallen, neuraesthenia (ME-like tiredness) has risen. The rise is more than enough to account for the decrease in anxiety consultations, but not quite enough to account for the decrease in consultations for depressive illness.

The upward trends in depressive behaviour are discernible worldwide. In Japan speculation relates it to work stress; in Hong Kong to overcrowding. It is most unlikely that this worldwide increase in despair could be put down to any one single factor. Just about every aspect of existence contributes to stress, as we have seen in chapter 8. Among the most important factors are:

1   economic problems – poverty and unemployment
2   reduced family support
3   the philosophy of individualism, leading to reduced social support
4   the decline of religion, with its spiritual and social support and its moral values
5   changing gender roles.
6   loss of sense of purpose.

The last point is inferred from the fact that suicide dropped markedly during the last war. Anecdotally, at least one person with clear manic depressive illness both before and after the war was completely stable during his time of service as a tank corporal during the war. The causes are thought to be a sense of social solidarity and a sense of a common enemy, leading to a sense of common purpose.

Only a fool would infer that what the world needs to put things right is therefore fighting a war; but the war model of social remediation does offer an insight into a possible solution. The 'enemy' for us today, the real threat to our security, is not some external state or ideology, but the social tensions generated by the divergence between rich and poor and the environmental threats to our long-term security from resource depletion, species loss, pollution, ozone imbalance, global warming and the rest. When war is declared on these conditions (as it must be in the long run, when the problems become so acute that politicians can no longer deny their existence), the economic mobilization, social cohesion and sense of purpose that will result will offer a substantive remedy to any of the ills that we now face. In the words of the old Chinese saying, the danger also gives us an opportunity.

The typical pattern of development in environmental knowledge is that causes are adopted first by patients and pressure groups, and dismissed as emotional scaremongering by medical, industrial and government authorities. This position persists for ten or 20 years, when emerging weight of evidence finally vindicates the environmentalists.

# THE OZONE LAYER — A PRECAUTIONARY TALE

The story of the destruction of the stratospheric ozone layer exemplifies this pattern. The first warnings that CFCs could catalyse the breakdown of stratospheric ozone came from American scientists Rowland and Molina in 1974. Environmentalists campaigned until the USA, Canada and Sweden banned the non-essential use of CFCs in 1979–80. Their campaign was discounted on the grounds that:

1   the concentrations of CFCs, being measured in parts per trillion, were too small to make any difference
2   even if the ozone layer were to become thinned, the resulting increased flux of ultraviolet light would create more ozone and therefore the problem would be self-curing.

Throughout the 1980s the production of CFCs continued more or less unabated until the British scientist Joe Farman discovered the ozone hole over the Antarctic in 1985. He might have published sooner had not the computer concerned with measuring the ozone levels suffered the same fault as the minds of many industrial and government scientists and dismissed its own readings as being too out of tune with its expectations to be true. Four years after Farman's paper in *Nature* , the first international agreement in Helsinki was reached, with the target of ceasing CFC production by the year 2000. Despite this and subsequent agreements, government refrigerators in morgues and munitions factories are still leaking out tens of thousands of tonnes of CFCs each year. Leakage repair of machinery replacement is not undertaken simply because it is not required by the international agreements.

The lesson to be learned from the ozone layer tragedy is that the precautionary principle must be applied rigorously, especially where potentially serious consequences are possible.

# IONIZING RADIATION

The term radiation covers a wide spectrum of energies from radio waves with a wavelength of more than a mile to gamma-rays with wavelengths of less than a micron and, confusingly, high-energy particles such as electrons, neutrons and helium nuclei. The major division to be made is between ionizing and non-ionizing radiation. In order to maintain some form of volume control in dealing with this huge field, this section will deal only with the assessment of health impacts on humans.

## Biological effects of ionizing radiation

Ionizing radiation can be subdivided simply into X-rays, gamma-rays and beta- and alpha-particles. X- and gamma-rays are highly penetrative forms of energy, which flood throughout the tissues as a ray of light passes through air. Beta-parti- cles are high-velocity electrons that release X-rays when they hit other matter. Alpha-rays are relatively heavy particles, and lay a denser track of ions behind them. To allow for this fact, a 'Q' factor of 20 is applied to alpha-radiation in for- mulae to calculate its biological effects. All forms affect biological tissues by creat- ing ions – electrically charged particles – as they pass through. This results in the creation of free radicals. Cells are most vulnerable to these effects when they are in the process of division. Therefore tissues which divide rapidly and constantly, such as the lining of the intestines, sperm and the blood-forming tissues, are more at risk from the effects of radiation.

If radiation hits a cell during the process of cell division, the DNA strands may be altered by the ions formed. There are three possible consequences of this impact.

1   The DNA is so damaged that the two daughter cells die.
2   The damage is slight and the cell repairs itself perfectly.
3   The damage is too great to be repaired perfectly, but not enough to be lethal. The daughter cells therefore continue to live on, but as mutants which, if they are not killed by the immune system, will form a cancer.

Busby[29] has posited a 'second event' mechanism that pushes outcome 2 towards outcome 3. If an isotope such as strontium-90 is incorporated into a chromosome, it will at some stage decay (half of it will decay within 29 years), releasing a burst of beta-radiation energy. Let us say that the damage so caused is reparable damage. However, in decaying, it has turned into yttrium-90, and half of that will decay again within three days. It is possible that the energy release in the second event may disrupt the cell reparation process, turning a repair event into a death or mutation event.

The importance of this is that the biological effects of radiation are far more complex than the simple rule of thumb methods of radiation safety modelling allow. The more we know about radiation, the lower the safe limit becomes.

Our knowledge of the biological effects of radiation (radiobiology) is based mainly on calculations of the doses received by the victims of the unnecessary bombing of Hiroshima and Nagasaki.[30]

This basis for the science of radiobiology has been criticized on various grounds.

1 The calculation had to be revised when an underground test showed that the bombs delivered a different dose from that which had been originally assumed.

2 The statistical method used has been criticized for using a single-sided test instead of double-sided.[31,32]

3 Masking effects have been underestimated.[33]

4 The study assumes that all of the effect came from the all-pervading gamma-radiation rather than radioisotopes which are taken into the body and deliver the dose from inside, often to specific tissues. It has been claimed[34] that an early study by the Japanese showed a four-fold increase in cancer rates among the survivors compared with controls who were unaffected by fallout.[35] By the time the Americans began their study, the control groups themselves were contaminated internally with radionuclides from fallout, which would have diminished the perceived effect of the radiation.

5 Petkau[36] has found evidence that very low-level radiation may be more damaging than hitherto expected because of the effect of free radicals on membranes.

6 The 'second event' effect quoted above may increase the biological effectiveness of radiation.

7 The behaviour of X- and gamma-rays in the body is quite distinct from that of radionuclides, which are carried to specific points in the body. For instance, plutonium and strontium are conducted to the bone, where they lie in close proximity to the blood-forming tissues. Iodine-131 is selectively taken up by the thyroid. Their effects on their target organs are therefore far greater than the simple physical measurement of their radioactivity would indicate.

From this it must be gathered that the 'gold standard' by which the biological effectiveness is judged is showing signs of verdigris, and scholastic arguments which dismiss possible effects on the grounds that insufficient radiation has been received to cause the unobserved effects (p. 148) are unjustified.

# The health effects of man-made radiation

Radiation in high doses is known to be a cause of cancer and birth deformities in humans. The question is 'does it appreciably affect the health of human populations in the doses produced by human activity?'. There is a vast literature on this subject, much of it steeped in controversy. What follows here is a distillation of the least controversial aspects.

1 Fallout from nuclear weapons tests in the 1950s and 1960s had measurable effects on the population of the world, and new aspects are still being evaluated. It is established that:

- infant mortality increased after atmospheric nuclear tests.[37] Low birthweight relates to the concentration of strontium-90 in bone.[38] The same study also

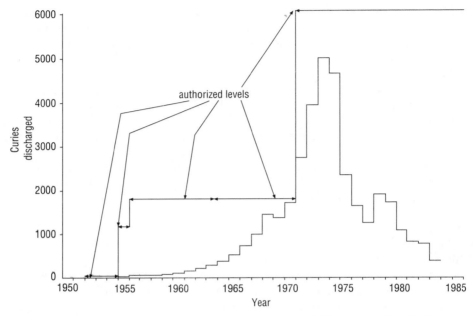

**Figure 11.3** Flexible discharge authorization limits from Sellafield. Source: The Black Report.

notes the rising incidence of pneumonia, septicaemia, cancer and AIDS in the 'baby boom' generation, and speculates that the explanation may be immune deficiency and increased pathogen mutations due to increased environmental radiation.
● Down's syndrome increased in areas of the UK affected by fallout.[39]

The effects of the nuclear industry should be divided into routine and accidental releases.

## Routine releases

Routine releases occur through the normal working of the plant. They are covered by licenses to release, although the limits set by the authorities are movable goal-posts, as can be seen in Figure 11.3, which shows that the authorized discharged limits were relaxed in order to legitimize the release of a larger quantity of radioactive waste. This is equivalent to widening the goalposts to accommodate a myopic striker whose team must always win.

Suggestive evidence for the effects of low-dose radiation is that leukaemia and other cancers are increased around the following sites around nuclear installations:

● Sellafield
● Trawsfynydd

- Dounreay
- Springfield
- Aldermaston
- Burghfield
- west coast of Scotland (affected by Hunterston and Chapelcross)
- Holy Loch (nuclear submarine base)
- Lydney (opposite Oldbury and Berkeley Nuclear Power Station)
- Lingen, Germany
- Rocky Flats, USA
- Savannah River, USA.

Although individually the analysis of each of these incidents may be criticized, collectively they form a picture of some risk to populations around some plants at least.

Against this evidence, the nuclear industry sets the pie chart of the dose to humans from various sources (Figure 11.4). Radioactive releases in this chart appear insignificant at 0.1% of the total. This presentation obscures the fact that the releases are not evenly spread throughout the population, but concentrated on those around the installations, who will show a larger segment of total input coming from emissions.

Martin Gardner has produced evidence that seemed to show that radiation workers have an increased risk of producing offspring with leukaemia, but subsequent research has not confirmed his findings.[40]

Kinlen has produced several papers which support his hypothesis that the clusters of childhood leukaemia observed around nuclear installations can be

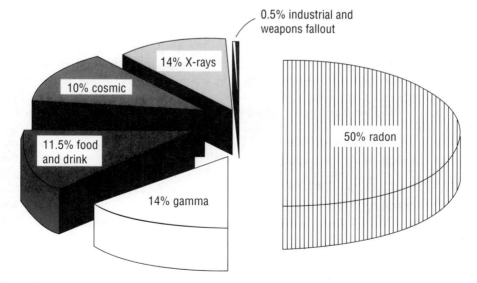

**Figure 11.4**  Radiation dose pie chart. Source: National Radiological Protection Board.

explained by the influx of workers from outside who import viruses which cause leukaemia.[41] Viruses are known to be able to cause leukaemia in cats, but no evidence exists of their ability to cause the disease in humans. Nevertheless, Kinlen has made a strong case that the influx of workers into an area may cause, through whatever reason, an increase in the local leukaemia rates. If this mechanism is generally accepted, it would follow that all large construction projects should pay a levy to the local health care services to cover the cost of treating the leukaemias that they will cause, and should also set aside money to pay compensation to individual sufferers.

The view put forward by the nuclear industry is that routine releases have no effect upon health. This hypothesis has not been tested by a prospective trial, that is one that goes forward in time, studying the health of people affected by the emissions, rather than retrospective trials, which look back at their health records.

The experiment to test the hypothesis would be designed in this way: the area around a nuclear installation would be surveyed for actual deposition of fallout attributable to emissions from the station. The population affected, or a representative sample, would have a close watch kept on their health, and some would have full blood tests. Milk from the area accepting fallout from the installation would be monitored, and the population drinking that milk would be noted. Meteorological conditions on days when large atmospheric releases were made would be assessed, and on at least one thermic day cumulus clouds that had taken up emissions would be tracked, and the radiological content of the cloud would be assessed. Only at the end of a study of this magnitude would we be able to know with certainty that routine emissions do not affect health.

## Accidental releases

The Chernobyl accident on 21 April 1986 was the worst nuclear accident the world has yet known. The release was equivalent to 10% of all the releases of nuclear weapons tests. It was the result of inherently unsafe design and negligent management: the engineers turned off a safety system to speed up a turbine experiment. Engineers in the UK assure us that it couldn't happen here (Figure 11.5). This assurance, which has long been a key argument of the British nuclear industry (which passed responsibility for the Windscale fire of 1958 on to the Ministry of Defence), has been severely damaged by the revelation that safety procedures were not followed when a crane part fell into a chute in the reactor at Trawsfynydd nuclear power station in Wales. This blocked the flow of coolant gas, and serious overheating of the affected fuel rod was only avoided because the part cracked the graphite case, allowing some gas to escape. Nine hours elapsed between the accident and reactor shutdown. Opinion is divided as to whether commercial considerations figured in the shutdown delay, and whether the accident could have led to a Chernobyl-type meltdown, but it is now undeniable that British reactor operators are capable of making serious errors.

Theoretical estimates of the expected effects of the release from the Chernobyl reactor vary from 5000 to 250 000 cancers worldwide. In theory, increased

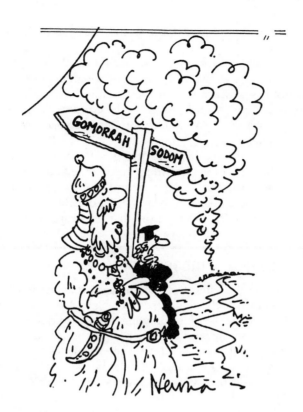

**Figure 11.5** 'Of course, it could never happen here…'. Source: Private Eye.

leukaemias in children are expected to occur from 1988–96 onwards, whereas other cancers will not begin to manifest themselves until the year 2006. In fact, Ukraine's health minister reports[42] that, by 1994, already 125 000 had died as a consequence of the accident. Many of these were involved in the clean-up operation. Sixty per cent of those who were children and adolescents at the time of the accident run the risk of thyroid cancer. A study[43] has shown that the incidence of childhood thyroid cancer is 62 times higher since Chernobyl. Children are more affected because they drink more milk (contaminated with iodine-131) and their thyroid glands are smaller. Children in the affected area also suffer more from diseases of the blood, digestive, respiratory and nervous systems.

The incidence of childhood leukaemia following Chernobyl has been studied in two papers published in the *BMJ* in 1994. Auvinen *et al.*[44] found an increase in the incidence of childhood leukaemia of one or two cases per year in the area with highest exposure up to 1992, but the numbers fell short of statistical significance. A Swedish study of cases from 1980 to 1992[45] found a similar non-statistically significant increase in acute lymphoblastic leukaemia in children under five years old. Both of these studies are somewhat premature, since the full harvest of leukaemia will not be gathered until 1996, so that they are underestimating the full numbers.

Down's syndrome, which is a chromosomal rather than a genetic defect, has been studied after Chernobyl, since its effect is apparent within a year of irradiation. An increase of cases was found in West Berlin.[46]

Infant mortality is affected, with livebirths reduced by 20% in Poland, and effects noticed in Germany and the USA. Adult mortality increased by 5.3% in the USA between May and August 1986.

The Russian nuclear industry has had the good fortune to get away with its error on a no-cost basis. Britain's farmers have received £10 million from the Ministry of Agriculture, Fisheries and Food, and the government, although it has said that it would seek compensation from Russia, clearly has no realistic expectation of succeeding in extracting money from that bankrupt economy.

# Nuclear insurance and compensation[47]

The academic debate on the effects of radiation on humans is infinitely complex, and seems set to continue indefinitely. Insurance against risk is one practical aspect of the matter which could be useful in drawing the whole diffuse field into focus.

Natural law dictates that, in any activity, humans must act responsibly, that is they must be able to be called to account for the results of their actions. If I drive recklessly in such a way that I kill a child, I must be called to account and be punished. If through no fault of my own I am involved in an accident and kill a child, the family of the injured child will rightly receive compensation from my insurance. If I drive without insurance cover, I am committing an offence and can expect to be punished.

Similarly, if, through a freak accident, the blade comes off a wind turbine and kills a child, the insurance policy of the owners of the wind turbine will pay compensation to the family. And if a sewage farm causes a pollution incident that kills fish in a river, the polluters will pay the anglers' society compensation to restock the river. These observations are commonplace and obvious.

It is therefore extremely surprising to discover that the nuclear industry does not have insurance cover sufficient to give full compensation to victims of its releases, routine or accidental. Instead, it has been granted a form of limited liability by the Standing Committee on Nuclear Liability, an international body whose remit is, ironically, the protection of the victims of nuclear accidents.

The setting of compensation for nuclear accidents is ferociously complex, involving international law (since pollution crosses state boundaries), and because there may be a delay of up to 30 years between the incident and the appearance of cancers caused by the accident. Factors to be covered include:

1   birth abnormalities
2   cancers
3   psychological trauma

4   environmental damage
5   loss of agricultural produce and land
6   loss of property
7   loss of profit and productivity
8   population evacuation and relocation
9   clean-up operations.

At least 12 estimates have been made of the cost of major nuclear accidents.[48] None of them attempts complete coverage of all the factors, and the results vary from a pusillanimous US$2 billion (French Ministry of Industry estimate for a release limited to 3–5% of Chernobyl) to a not inconsiderable DM83.2 trillion or, US$60 trillion.

The revenue in 1990 for OECD nuclear electricity sales was US$109 billion, so that a 10% levy to cover accident liability would yield $10 billion per year, which over ten years would build up to a kitty of more than $100 billion. James Asseltine of the US Nuclear Regulatory Commission gave a probability of one Chernobyl-type accident every 5–20 years for a complement of 490 nuclear reactors world-wide.[49] This levy therefore gives a modest and conservative start to the process of instituting full compensation to victims of any future nuclear accidents. It should be instituted without delay, and the figure adjusted as and when more accurate assessments of the damage emerge. Not to do so would be to violate the polluter pays principle and to keep artificially low the market price of nuclear energy. It would also impose further burdens on the health services budget, effectively forcing it to subsidize nuclear power.

# Non-ionizing radiation[50]

Non-ionizing radiation or electromagnetic fields (EMFs) are radiations with wave-lengths longer than that of light that do not form ions in the tissues they affect. Assessment of their health effects is a difficult science, and debate is marked by profound disagreement between those who are convinced of health risks and other scientists, both independent and those employed by the electrical power industries, who are not so convinced.

It is possible to have an electric field without a magnetic field, but not vice versa. All live wires bear an electric field whether or not they are in use. Once an appliance is switched on and the current flows, the magnetic field comes into play. In most studies, the magnetic field only is recorded, because it is easier to measure.

The controversies surrounding EMFs reflect the complexity of the physics and biology of the subject. The effect of the radiation is influenced by:

1   topography
2   wavelength
3   frequency

4  directionality
5  balance
6  synergy
7  ionization of ambient air
8  confounding factors.

Topographical features include natural sources of EMF, including groundwater flows (which induce natural electric fields), natural fluctuations of the Earth's magnetic field, and piezoelectricity, which occurs as a result of stresses in the Earth's mantle.

Wavelengths and frequency may have specific effects on specific tissues. For example, the human skull resonates at the frequencies of radio waves from portable telephones. Coghill suggests that exposure to microwaves may induce myeloid leukaemia, whereas exposure to power frequencies may induce lymphocytic leukaemia.[50]

Directionality – the predominant direction of the current – may mean that fields that have bias set in one direction may be more biologically effective than fields which vary or alternate.

The EMF is balanced when the neutral wire is adjacent to the live wire and carrying the same current. If the neutral is connected to earth, the electrical field may be much larger than expected.

Synergy may occur between EMF and other physical or chemical agents with a tendency to produce the same end effects. Synergy may also operate between the electrical and magnetic components of any one field, and many studies are inadequate because only the magnetic field is measured.

Ionization of ambient air is thought by some to have a variety of effects on allergies, headaches and sense of well-being, positive ions being associated with problems and negative ions being associated with health. It must be said that because of extravagant claims from the manufacturers of ionizers, the topic has been relegated to the fringes of science; nevertheless, there is a body of evidence that is enough at least to merit more research.

Confounding factors include the common factors in assessing the health risks borne by any population, together with the possibility that high electromagnetic fields may also increase the amount of ionizing radiation in the area.

## Effects of EMF

Many effects have been associated with EMF, from miscarriage through cot deaths and AIDS to ME, and controversy continues to surround many of the claims, some of which are not subjected to any standards of causality. The consistent effects to emerge from studies are neoplasia ('cancer') and depression.

### Neoplasia

Neoplasia has been associated with EMF in several studies, which are summarized in Table 11.1.

**Table 11.1** Neoplasia and EMF

| Study group | Source of radiation (researcher) | Finding |
| --- | --- | --- |
| Children | LuaLuaLei, Hawaii – US Navy Communications[50] | Fourfold increase in cancer |
| General population | Gibraltar – communications[50] | Cancer increase |
| Soldiers | Unknown – Szmigielski *et al.*[51] | Sevenfold increase in cancer |
| Three hundred and thirty-four childhood cancer patients | US domestic wiring – Wertheimer and Leeper[52] | Twofold increased likelihood of living near electrical wiring installations |
| Childhood cancer patients | 200 kV power lines (Tomenius,[53] Sweden) | Twofold increased likelihood of living <25 m from line |
| US Embassy staff, Moscow | KGB microwaves – 4 mW/cm$^2$ [54] | High cancer levels |
| Children | Voice of America transmitters, Delano, CA | Thirteen cancers |

Given the results in Table 11.1, why is there so little concern on the part of government? The National Radiological Protection Board (NRPB) case[55] is that experimental evidence shows that EMF of the type created by proximity to some power lines can affect electroencephalogram patterns, the ability to perform complex reasoning and the output of melatonin from the pineal gland. The last may affect mood and cancer formation. Experiments also showed effects on osteoblasts (bone-forming cells), RNA and cell protein transcription. Throughout, only consistent results are considered: occasional results that are not reproduced are not considered. Epidemiological evidence has been reviewed by an Advisory Group on Non-ionising Radiation under the chairmanship of Sir Richard Doll. It considered eight studies, including those of Wertheimer and Leeper and Tomenius, and concluded that they provided 'weak evidence in support of the postulated association between EMF and cancer, especially brain cancer and leukaemia'.[56] Since the Group reported, a further large and well-designed study of occupational groups in Canada and France[57] has shown a higher risk for non-lymphoid leukaemia, especially acute myeloid leukaemia, in electrical workers. Finally, three Scandinavian studies have been pooled[58] and shown a doubled risk of leukaemia for children living close to power lines. The NRPB Assistant Director could not deny this doubling; instead he presented it as a 'very small increase' since only 13 cases were involved, presumably a 'price worth paying' in the interests of cheap electricity.

Overall, the attitude of the NRPB is that electromagnetic radiation is, like a human with civil rights, innocent until proved guilty. It also appears to be unaware of the precautionary principle, since it specifically refuses to commit itself even to advising against building new houses under existing power lines. It is hard to avoid the conclusion that the NRPB as presently constituted sees its task as that of protecting radiation from people, rather than people from radiation.

The old Central Electricity Generating Board's research budget into EMF was £500 000. The advertising budget for electricity privatization was £100 000 000.

It is too early to put a cost on the impact of EMF on the NHS's cancer spending. The number of people living under power lines is not great, and so the number of cases of leukaemia caused is probably fewer than 1–2 per year.

## Depression

The experimental data accepted by the NRPB above indicate that reasoning, EEG patterns and melatonin output may be affected by EMF. There is much evidence to show that people exposed to EMF may become depressed.

1   People living near high electrical fields have a high incidence of depression[59] and suicide.[60]
2   Out of 23 British microwave scientists who have died, seven committed suicide and 13 may have done so.
3   Suicide among scientists at Marconi (microwave communications) is twice the average.

In conclusion, the science of EMF is phenomenally complex, and we do not yet have enough data to put a price on the impact. There is enough evidence, however, to put a levy on electrical power and goods in order to pay for further research.

# DENTAL MERCURY

Mercury is a toxic heavy metal, which at occupational levels of exposure has been associated with tumours of lung, kidney and the central nervous system.[61] Mercury is a component of dental amalgam, and it is known that mercury vapour is released during chewing, and in much greater amounts during replacement of dental fillings – in fact, this is the greatest source of general human exposure. Air-borne mercury may be a problem around crematoria, due to the burning of fillings,[62] (11 kg/year may be released from one crematorium chimney). Dentists should have mercury traps fitted to their waste water systems to prevent pollution of sewage sludge – and to save a valuable resource.

In the mouth mercury may be a causal factor in gum disease and lichen planus, a troublesome hypersensitivity reaction in the lining of the mouth.[63] In rats mercury may affect nerve membrane structure, and in monkeys amalgam may help produce antibiotic-resistant bacteria in the gut.[64]

There therefore appears to be a case for amalgam to answer. In the meantime, it is not advisable for people who are worried about their fillings to request total replacement, as the drilling is thought to create a larger dose of mercury than day-to-day chewing. It does seem reasonable, however, to request that as and when fillings become due for replacement, this should be with non-mercury material. There is a white, light-cured plastic available which is serviceable, although not quite so durable as amalgam; but no one yet knows the long-term effects of this plastic, so there is a choice to be made.

---

### Recommendation

Alternatives to mercury should be available on the NHS.

---

# FLUORIDE

Under the 1985 Water Fluoridation Act fluoride may be added to drinking water in the UK at the request of the regional health authority. At present, 11% of drinking water in the UK is treated. Most untreated water usually contains a background level of fluoride of about 0.1 mg/l, although levels of more than 1 mg/l are occasionally found; the Act permits levels of up to 1 mg/l. The low level of take-up is partly due to an interesting little bureaucratic quirk: the boundaries of regional health authorities are not the same as those of water companies, so that if a health authority decides to treat it may be illegally affecting supplies of people in a neighbouring health authority.

Dentists are agreed that fluoride added to drinking water reduces the incidence of dental caries (decay). The incidence of caries is 50% higher in water regions which are very low in fluoride, and the introduction of fluoride has been shown to decrease caries, whereas its withdrawal has been shown to increase caries.

Campaigners opposed to fluoridation[a] argue that:

1  it represents mass medication, and is therefore an infringement of civil liberties
2  it is introduced chiefly because it is a convenient way for the chemical industry to rid itself of a toxic by-product
3  it may induce fluorosis (speckled discoloration) of teeth
4  it may be associated with unwanted side-effects, namely bone disorders, Down's syndrome, cancer and skeletal fluorosis.

The mass medication argument also applies to chlorine, which is added to prevent infection, and also carries a health risk. However, it could be argued that in the case of chlorine, it is the water which is being medicated, not the consumer. Individuals who are still troubled by this point can invest in a water filter to remove both additives, although this is an enforced expenditure. The other health gains would make filter purchase an effective use of money.

[a] National Pure Water Association, 17 Sycamore Lane, West Bretton, Wakefield WF4 4JR.

The by-product argument may well be true, but is offset by the benefit argument. It is a good green principle to find a use for all 'waste products', so the origin of the fluoride, and the economics of its use, are of marginal importance, although there is some evidence of truth bending in the history of the campaign for fluoridation in the USA, which is regrettable.

The dental fluorosis argument is essentially cosmetic, and cosmetic benefits of having a number of people with teeth discoloured by caries needs to be set against the advantages of having a number of people with teeth discoloured by fluoridation. A detailed accounting exercise would help to settle this equation.

The side-effect argument is therefore the key to the debate. Is there good evidence of harm, and how does the side-effect balance with the desired end effect?

First, it may be argued that the dose is somewhat disproportionate, as only one gallon in every 2500 is consumed by children, who are the target of the medication. Furthermore, bottle-fed infants may be overdosed, since the fluoride is concentrated in their feeds. Some brands tested in the USA show varying levels of between 0.26 ppm and 3.98 ppm fluoride. If these are made up with fluoridated water at 1 ppm an infant could be swallowing almost 5 ppm of fluoride per litre of milk. Commercial juices and strained meals, plus toothpaste swallowed by older infants, would add even more fluoride, so that there is a danger that guidelines could be exceeded.

In 1959 Dr Janel Rapaport at the University of Wisconsin found a statistical connection between fluoridated drinking water and Down's syndrome. He found that in non-fluoridated communities the incidence of this condition was 34 per 100 000 and in fluoridated towns it was 72 per 100 000. The number of people studied was one-third of a million. These findings were published in *The Bulletin of the National Academy of Medicine* in France.

In 1965 Dr Alfred Taylor at the University of Texas showed that mice develop cancer at an earlier age on fluoridated water. A total of 645 mice were used. He also found that four of the mice on fluoridated water developed bladder stones – a condition never before observed in his mouse colony. It is interesting that the fluoride content of some human bladder stones has been found to be 1500–1700 ppm.

Only half the fluoride we ingest is excreted by our kidneys – the rest is deposited in our bones. This fluoride may lead to skeletal fluorosis, which resembles arthritis in its early clinical stages. Patients experience pain and stiffness of joints and movement is restricted. Radiographic examination will disclose osteosclerosis. Clinically significant skeletal fluorosis occurs when there is natural fluoride present in water supplies, mostly below 2.5 ppm.

In conclusion, it appears that there is at least a case to answer on the subject of fluoride. It is an effective agent for stopping dental caries, but the savings need to be set against the costs in terms of Down's syndrome risk, skeletal and dental fluorosis and possibly cancer. While so many doubts remain, it would be foolish to press on with mass medication, especially since regulation of sugar content in food and a polluter pays tax on sugar could achieve the same end.

# CONCLUSION

Environmental agents are very numerous; they interact, they produce subtle effects which are difficult to distinguish from the background 'noise' of illness. There are more than 60 000 potential agents of ill-health in our physical environment. Socioeconomic conditions are fourfold: unemployment, poor housing, social breakdown and poverty. Whereas socioeconomic conditions have been known to affect health for a century or more, awareness of the effects of the environment on our health is barely accepted in some quarters where the conservative mindset prevails, and is actively resisted in quarters where investigation and regulation of environmental agents might adversely affect profits even though, as has been shown, the nation as a whole would be more prosperous as well as healthier if the economy were to be guided into socially and environmentally beneficial pathways. In the next and final chapter, we shall assess the bills of health by looking at the cost of these conditions to the NHS, and by looking at some of the reforming bills that would have to go through parliament to bring about a healthier nation.

# REFERENCES

1   Robertson C F, Heycock E, Bishop J *et al.* (1991) Prevalence of asthma in Melbourne School Children: changes over 26 years. *BMJ*: **302**; 1116–8

2   Hahhtela T, Linholm H, Bjorksten F *et al.* (1990) Prevalence of asthma in Finnish young men. *BMJ*: **301**; 266–8.

3   Rusznak C, Devalia J L, Herdman M J *et al.* (1994) The effect of six hours' exposure to 400 ppb nitrogen dioxide and/or 200 ppb sulphur dioxide on inhaled allergen response in mild asthmatic subjects. *Clin Exp Allergy*: **24**; 166.

4   Newman Taylor A (1995) Environmental determinants of asthma. *Lancet*: **345**; 296–9.

5   Austin J B, Russell G, Adam M G *et al.* (1994) Prevalence of asthma and wheeze in the Highlands of Scotland. *Arch Dis Child*: **71**; 211–6.

6   Burroughs B, Hallonen M, Barbee R A *et al.* (1981) The relationship of serum immunoglobulin E to cigarette smoking. *Am Rev Respir Dis*: **124**; 523–5.

7   Bromey P G, Chinh S, Rona R J (1990) Has the prevalence of asthma increased in children? Evidence from the national study of health and growth. *BMJ*: 300; 1306–10.

8   Read C (1994) *How Vehicle Pollution Affects our Health*. The Ashden Trust, London.

9   Von Mutius E, Fritzch C, Weiland S W *et al.* (1992) Prevalence of asthma and allergic disorders among children in united Germany: a descriptive comparison. *BMJ*: **305**; 1395–9.

10    Magnussen H, Jones R, Nowak D (1993) Effect of air pollution on the prevalence of asthma and allergy: lessons from the German reunification. *Thorax*: **48**; 879–81.

11    Smoke in the streets: the rising impact of dirty diesels (1991) *Clean Air* (Journal of the Nation's Society for Clean Air): **21(2)**; 53–60.

12    Ishizaki T, Koizumi K, Ikemori R *et al.* (1987) Studies of prevalence of Japanese cedar pollinosis among residents in a densely cultivated area. *Ann Allergy*: **58**; 265–70.

13    Miamoto T, Takafuji S, Tadokoro A *et al.* (1988) Allergy and changing environments – industrial/urban pollution. In: W Pichler, B M Staedler, C Dakinden *et al.* (eds) *Progress in Allergy and Clinical Immunology*. Hoj Refe and Huber, Toronto. pp. 256–70.

14    Berciano F A, Crespo M, Bao C G *et al.* (1987) Serum levels of total IgE in non-allergic children: influence of genetic and environmental factors. *Allergy*: **42**; 276–83.

15    Meredith S R, Taylor U M, McDonald J C (1991) Occupational respiratory disease in United Kingdom 1989. A report to the British Thoracic Society of Occupational Medicine by the SWORD project group. *Br J Ind Med*: **48**; 292–8.

16    Schwartz J, Dockery D W (1992) Particulate air pollution and daily mortality in Steubenville, Ohio. *Am J Epidemiol*: **135**; 12–19.

17    Schwartz J, Slater D, Larson T V *et al.* (1992) Particulate air pollution and hospital emergency room visits for asthma in Seattle. *Am Rev Respir Dis*: **145(4 part 2)**; 88.

18    Jaakola J K, Paunio M, Virtanen M *et al.* (1991) Low level air pollution and upper respiratory infections in children. *Am J Public Health*: **81**; 1060–3.

19    Presentation to Socialist Medical Society, Manchester.

20    Seaton A, Godden D J, Brown K (1994) Increase in asthma: a more toxic environment or a more susceptible population? *Thorax*: **49**; 171–4.

21    Letter. *Aust NZ J Med*: December 1994.

22    de Cock J, Westveer K, Heederick D *et al.* (1994) Time to pregnancy and occupational exposure to pesticides in fruit growers in The Netherlands. *Occup Environ Med*: **51**; 693–9.

23    Shane B S and Gutenmann W H (1993) Variability over time in the mutagenicity of ashes from municipal solid-waste incinerators. *Mutat Res*: **301**; 39–43.

24    Gough M (1991) Human health effects: what the data indicate. *Sci Total Environ*: **104**; 129–58.

25    Raloff J (1993) Ecocancers: do environmental factors underlie a breast cancer epidemic? *Sci News*: **144**; 10–13.

26    Thornton J (1992) *Breast Cancer and the Environment: The Chlorine Connection*. Greenpeace, London.

27    Cowan L D, Gordis L, Tonascia J A *et al.* (1981) Breast cancer incidence in women with progesterone deficiency. *Am J Epidemiol*: **114**; 209–17.

28   OPCS (1994) *Survey of Psychiatric Morbidity.* HMSO, London.

29   Busby C C (1995) *Wings of Death: Nuclear Pollution and Human Health.* Green Audit Books, Aberystwyth.

30   Alperowitz G (1990) Why the United States dropped the bomb. *Technol Rev:* Aug/Sept.

31   Bland J M (1994) Statistical analysis inappropriate (letter). *BMJ:* **208**; 339.

32   Darby S C, Doll R, Kendall G M (1994) Authors' reply, (letters). *BMJ:* **208**; 339.

33   Stewart A M (1982) Delayed effects of A-bomb radiation: A review of recent mortality rates and risk estimates for five year survivors. *J Epidemiol Commun Health:* **35**; 80–6.

34   Busby C (1994) *Radiation and Cancer in Wales.* Green Audit Wales, Aberystwyth.

35   Harada T and Ishida M (1961) First Report of the Research Comittee on Tumour Statistics, Hiroshima City Medical Association, Japan. *J Nat Cancer Inst:* **29**; 1253–64.

36   Petkau A (1980) Radiation effects from a membrane perspective. *Acta Physiol Scand:* **492 (suppl.)**; 81–90.

37   Gould J W and Goldman B A (1990) *Deadly Deceit: Low-level Radiation, High-level cover up.* Four Walls Eight Windows, New York.

38   Gould J M and Sternglass E J (1994) Nuclear fallout, low birth-weight and immune deficiency. *Int J Health Services:* **24**; 311–35.

39   Bound J, Francis B, Harvey P (1995) *J Epidemiol Community Health:* **49**; 164–70.

40   Gardner M J, Hall A J, Downes S *et al.* (1987) Follow-up Study of Children Born to Workers Resident in Seascale, West Cumbria. *BMJ:* **295**; 819–21.

41   Kinlen L J (1988) Evidence for Infective Cause of Childhood Leukaemia: Comparison of a Scottish New Town with Nuclear Reprocessing Sites in Britain. *Lancet:* **ii**; 1123–7.

42   ITAR-TASS newsagency 25 April 1995. Moscow, Russia.

43   Abelin T, Egger M, Ruchti C (1994) Belarus increase was probably caused by Chernobyl. *BMJ:* **309**; 1298.

44   Auvinen A, Hakama M, Arvela H *et al.* (1994) Fallout from Chernobyl and incidence of childhood leukaemia in Finland, 1976–92. *BMJ:* **309**; 151–4.

45   Hjalmars U, Kulldorf M, Gustafsson G (1994) Risk of acute childhood leukaemia in Sweden after the Chernobyl reactor accident. *BMJ:* **309**; 154–7.

46   Sperling K, Pelz J, Wegner R D *et al.* (1994) Significant increase in trisomy 21 in Berlin nine months after the Chernobyl reactor incident: temporal correlation or causal relation? *BMJ:* **309(6948)**; 158–62.

47   Greenpeace International (1994) Full Compensation for Nuclear Damage. Submission to 10th session of the SCNL of the International Atomic Energy Agency. Greepeace International, London.

48   Greenpeace International (1994) Review of estimates of the costs of major nuclear accidents. Submission to the 9th Session of the Standing Committee on Nuclear

Liability of the International Atomic Energy Agency. Greenpeace International, London.

49 Geiger J H (1992) Letter. *JAMA*: **257(2)**; 190–1.

50 Coghill R (1990) *Electropollution*. Thorsons, Wellingborough.

51 Szmigielski S, Bielec M *et al.* (1988) Immunologic and cancer-related aspects of exposure to low-level microwave and radio frequency fields. In: *Modern Bioelectricity*. Marcel Dekker, New York. pp. 861–925.

52 Wertheimer N, Leeper E (1979) Electrical wiring configurations and childhood cancer. *Am J Epidemiol*; **109**; 273–84.

53 Tomenius L (1986) 50 Hz electromagnetic environment and the incidence of childhood tumours in Stockholm County. *BEMS*: **7**; 191–207.

54 Becker R and Seldon G (1985) *The Body Electric: Electromagnetism and the Foundation of Life*. Morrow, New York.

55 Stather J, paper presented to NSCA 61st Conference October 1994.

56 Advisory Group of Non-ionising Radiation (1992) Electromagnetic fields and the risk of cancer. *Doc. NRPB*: **3(1)**; 1–138.

57 Theriault G, Goldberg M *et al.* (1994) Cancer risk associated with occupational exposure to electromagnetic fields among electric utility workers in Ontario and Quebec, Canada and France: 1970–1989. *Am J Epidemiol*: **139**; 550–72.

58 Ahlbohm A and Feychting M (1993) Electromagnetic fields and childhood cancer (letter). *Lancet*: **342**; 1295–6.

59 Perry F S and Pearl L (1988) Health effects of ELF fields and illness in multistorey blocks. *Public Health*: **102**; 11–18.

60 Perry F S, Reichmanis *et al.* (1981) Environmental power frequency magnetic fields and suicide. *Health Phys*: **41**; 267–77.

61 Bofetts P, Merler E, Vainio H (1993) Carcinogenicity of mercury and mercury compounds. *Scand J Work Environ Health*: **19**; 1–7.

62 Mills A (1990) Mercury and crematorium chimneys (letter). *Nature*: **346**; 615.

63 Swartzendruber D E (1993) The possible relationship between mercury from dental amalgam and diseases. I. Effects within the oral cavity. *Med Hypotheses*: **41**; 31–4.

64 Lorscheider F L, Vimy M J, Summers A O *et al.* (1995) The dental amalgam mercury controversy – inorganic mercury and the CNS; genetic linkage of mercury and antibiotic resistances in intestinal bacteria. *Toxicology*: **97**; 19–22.

# 12

# Bills of health

*The purpose of Government is to protect the vulnerable against exploitation by the powerful.*

Anon

This chapter gathers the cost to the NHS of unemployment, poverty, inadequate housing and environmental conditions and sets out some of the major parliamentary bills which are needed to bring about positive changes in the health of the nation. The figures are brought together here from other parts of the text for convenience.

## COUNTING UP THE DAMAGE

### Costs to the State

Where it is possible, it is interesting to include the cost to the nation as a whole. The following costs of unemployment (for 1994) are by no means comprehensive.

|  | £ million |
|---|---|
| Benefits to unemployed | 10 816 |
| Extra disablement | 4004 |
| Administration | 640 |
| Taxes foregone |  |
| Direct | 4581 |
| National insurance contributions | 3371 |
| Indirect taxes | 3164 |
| Total | £26 576 000 000 |

Source: Piachaud.[1]

Mortality due to unemployment adds another £4 119 000 000, so that the full cost to the state of unemployment is about £31 billion, or about 5% of the GDP.

It will be recalled that the total cost of asthma to the state (p. 219) is £1 billion per year. An estimate of the total cost to the state of the conditions covered in this book might prove very worthwhile.

# Costs to the health service

| Item | £ million |
|---|---|
| **Unemployment** | |
| GP consultations | 37.324 |
| Extra prescriptions | 19.194 |
| Lost prescription charges | 17.259 |
| Families of unemployed: consultations | 48.521 |
| Pharmaceutical bill for the families | 21.387 |
| Redundancy consultations | 1.969 |
| Pharmaceutical bill (redundancy) | 1.019 |
| Outpatient attendances | 116.800 |
| Dependents, increased outpatient attendance | 116.480 |
| Parasuicide (unemployment) | 21.770 |
| Inadequate housing | 2000.000 |
| Deprivation | 957.831 |
| **Environment** | |
| *Salmonella* infection increase due to global warming | 0.012 |
| Waterborne disease due to global warming | 0.050 |
| *Shigella sonnei* dysentery due to global warming | 0.059 |
| Natural medicines loss | 26.000 |
| Fish stocks depletion | 272.000 |
| Due to loss of the ozone shield | 7.700 |
| Population | 30.000 |
| Militarism | 3.000 |
| Trident | 500.000 |
| Lead | 2.700 |
| Aluminium | 2.700 |
| Synthetic perfumes | 6.800 |
| Chlorine | 9.230 |
| Asthma | 450.000 |
| Radon | 3.900 |
| Caffeine | 72.600 |
| Drug abuse    (high estimate) | 55.020 |
|                    (low estimate) | 38.650 |
| Occupational ill-health    (high) | 450.000 |
|                    (low) | 100.000 |
| Transport – heart disease | 82.300 |
|                    accidents | 320.000 |
| Food poisoning | 31.100 |
| Obesity    (high) | 1500.000 |
|                    (low) | 194.600 |
| Hyperactivity | 7.250 |
| Industrial air pollution | 85.500 |
| Pesticides | 14.000 |
| **Total**    (high estimate) | 7126.875 |
|                    (low estimate) | 5254.505 |

The total cost for identifiable annual treatment costs for diseases caused by conditions which could be prevented by resolute government action therefore lies between 5.2 and 7.1 billion pounds.

Taking the 1992 estimated annual budget of £35 408 000 000, and subtracting management costs of £1 045 000 000 gives an NHS clinical (patient care) budget of £34 362 900 000. Therefore between 15.3% and 20.7% of NHS clinical spending could be saved if the social, economic and environmental problems covered in this book were to be rectified.

The health-destroying conditions – unemployment, deprivation, inadequate housing and environmental pollution – have been worsening over the last few decades. Therefore their burden on the NHS is outstripping the increases in NHS funding, so that the net effect is that the NHS is becoming poorer – which bears out the claims of doctors and health service workers mentioned at the beginning.

Many other conditions have been omitted simply because it has not yet been possible to quantify the impact on health. Social conditions – lack of social support and integration, and a sense of powerlessness, together with the disruption of communities by agents as diverse as traffic, TV, videos, and the cult of individualism – are known to have a significant effect on health, but the effect cannot be quantified. Similarly, the strain on our immune systems imposed by new pollutants and stress (including noise-induced stress) creates a pool of illness which cannot be counted.

Other growing costs to the NHS not dealt with in this book include the ageing population, new and expensive medical technologies, lifestyle factors, growing patient demand and expectation (fuelled by the Patient's Charter), the growing pharmaceutical bill, and iatrogenic (i.e. side-effects of treatment) illnesses. Taken all together, these factors amount to an impressive change in the financial climate under which the NHS operates.

The total of £7.8 billion is a not inconsiderable sum. Any minister of health who arranged to increase the NHS annual budget by this amount would be hailed as a saviour of the service. Waiting lists would plummet, and quality of service would flourish gratifyingly. Front-line workers could devote themselves wholeheartedly to health promotional activities. Yet the same benefit is available not by increasing financial resource availability to the NHS, but by effecting beneficial reforms to the economic and social structure of the country which would also benefit the morale and financial stability of the people as a whole.

# ACHIEVING HEALTH OF THE NATION GOALS

The five key areas identified in the Health of the Nation project are:

1   coronary heart disease and stroke
2   cancers

3   mental illness
4   HIV/AIDS and sexual health
5   accidents.

Each of these areas is susceptible to improvement by political reforms.

## Coronary heart disease and stroke

### Recommendations

- tax sugars and saturated fats
- ban tobacco advertising
- improve exercise by providing cycleways.

## Cancers

### Recommendations

- ban tobacco advertising
- fund research into environmental carcinogens using pollution taxes
- regulate, restrict, tax and/or ban known carcinogens.

## Mental illness

### Recommendations

- end unemployment using wage subsidy
- improve social conditions with a programme of investment in community works and workers
- attack violence on the streets by improved social and economic equity, and by taxing violence on TV, film and videos.

## HIV/AIDS and sexual health

### Recommendations

- fund educational programmes adequately
- ban environmental pornography.

## Accidents

### Recommendations

- restrict speed of road transport
- increase the educational budget of the Department of Transport Accident Prevention Section.
- create safe havens on residential streets where pedestrians and children have legal priority over the motor car
- improve general social and economic conditions for the poorest sections of society
- review and redesign social housing to create a safer physical environment.

## PARLIAMENTARY BILLS

Parliamentary bills consist of 95% necessary legal verbiage and 5% content. The effect of the bills is set out below. These bills do not claim to be final or complete, but form the basis for bills which can be worked out by interested non-governmental organizations in cooperation with a reforming government, or for adoption by a majority of MPs in a cross-party consensus, as was the case with the Home Energy Conservation Bill.

## Wage Subsidy Bill

Parliament will abolish the 100% marginal taxation that is currently applied to benefits at the point when a claimant finds employment.

This bill enables the minister for employment to invite enterprises, whether public or private, existing or projected, to make application for the facility to take into their workforce new workers whose wages will be subsidized by their ability to retain their benefits while in employment – hereinafter called the wage subsidy scheme. Favoured schemes will include:

1 energy conservation
2 renewable energy technologies
3 energy-efficient goods manufacture
4 pollution control technology
5 waste minimization
6 repair
7 recycling
8 water management

9   sustainable agriculture
10  forestry and timber use
11  countryside management
12  housing – new building and refurbishment
13  improvements to the visual environment
14  public transport
15  education and training
16  counselling, caring and healing
17  community work
18  leisure and tourism
19  innovation, research and development
20  any business which passes a certain threshold in its environmental audit.

Successful employers will satisfy certain criteria to show that the product of the enterprise that will benefit from wage subsidy is:

● of benefit to society and/or to the environment
● is an investment, capable of a payback in social, ecological or financial terms.

Successful employers will accept certain conditions, namely:

● random unscheduled inspections of their books and working conditions
● they will undertake not to displace existing workers as they take on wage subsidy workers
● they will undertake to top up the state subsidy of the wage subsidy workers to an agreed minimum wage (if this is put in place) or to the normal market wage for the job, whichever is the greater.

# Housing Finance Bill

Parliament will abolish the Treasury accounting convention wherein the total cost of a new unit of accommodation built by public finance is shown in the public sector borrowing requirement for that year.

The minister for the environment shall empower local authorities to mobilize their capital receipts funds for housebuilding by:

1   giving low or zero-interest loans to self-help groups to enable them to re-furbish and build houses for themselves
2   giving to local authorities the power to issue Empty Property Use Orders to the owner(s) of any property that has been void for more than six months unless it can be shown that the owner has concrete plans for the use of that property in the next two months.

## Pollution Taxes (Restitution) Bill

This bill will give the Treasury the right, after due consideration by expert commit-
tees constituted for the purpose, to apply taxes to specified industrial processes at
specified points in the process, the taxes thus generated to be hypothecated to
research into, and remedying of, any effects of that process on human health or
the integrity of the environment. Producers will thereby accept full cradle-to-grave
responsibility for the effects of their product on the social and physical environment. The taxes will be set at a level that is sufficient for research and/or remediation to be carried out in full. For example:

- taxes raised on confectionery wrappers, cigarette packets and newspapers will
  be hypothecated to local authority street cleansing services
- taxes on hi-fi equipment will be hypothecated to local authority environmental
  health noise pollution services.

## Resource Taxation Bill

This bill will phase out taxation on employment (national insurance contributions
and lower rate income taxation), beginning with enterprises that have qualified
under the criteria above, and replace it with taxation applied to the use of scarce
and finite resources.

## European Union

It must be added that European Union law has to some extent removed the power
of parliament to do all that is necessary for the benefit of our people. It might
therefore be necessary to carry these bills, or some of them, through a European
parliament suitably empowered to enact this sort of legislation. This need not necessarily hold up progress since Europe is more advanced in its thinking than the
UK on environmental and social issues. The Netherlands, in particular, is far more
advanced in its public debate about the citizen's income than the UK.

## CONCLUSION

This book does not claim to be exhaustively scholarly or scientific – if it had been
it would never have been completed. It claims merely to take an overview of the
five major influences on the Health of the Nation and to focus their effects by considering them in terms of their costs on the National Health Service. Further work
over the years will refine, and in all probability increase our appreciation of, these

costs. Although research into the effects of external conditions on health is valuable, rational political action to improve health is more valuable still. Research should stimulate political action, not hold it back.

Years ago, a sailing ship was in difficulties off the coast of South America. Water supplies had run out and the crew were suffering sorely from thirst. They signalled another ship for water, which replied, 'drop a bucket over the side'. It was found that they were sailing in fresh water discharged from the Amazon.

We are like that ship. Unemployment causes poverty and social breakdown. It stresses the people affected and it stresses the economy as a whole. Unemployment is the water on which we sail – the basic assumption. By changing our assumptions about the situation, the danger becomes an opportunity. Unemployment is the key to resolving the many problems that we face. The 'unemployed' are not a problem, just an unused human resource. We need to lower the notional bucket and take them on board to help in the cooperative effort to create health in every sense – physical, mental, social, economic and spiritual.

In spite of all appearances, there is room for hope.

## REFERENCE

1    Piachaud D (1994) *A Price worth Paying?* Employment Policy Institute Economic Papers. Vol 8, No. 6.

# Glossary

**Antibody** The large Y-shaped protein molecules secreted by lymphocytes which attach themselves to antigens.

**Antigen** Any substance that is capable of provoking a reaction from the immune system.

**Aquifer** Underground watercourse.

**Benzodiazepines** Family of tranquillizing drugs, of which Valium and Librium are the best known.

**Carcinogen** Agent capable of causing cancer.

**Cohort studies** Studies that follow a group or groups of individuals over a period of time.

**Cross-sectional studies** Studies that examine the prevalence of disease in an area of several areas. These are useful for showing up 'snapshot' associations, but need to be checked against **longitudinal studies**.

**Ecological studies** Studies that use data which are routinely collected for statistical purposes, for instance disease rates, mortality rates and pollution levels.

**Environmental health officers (EHOs)** Local authority officers responsible for health matters in shops and public places and some forms of pollution.

**Field studies** See **Panel studies**.

**Genotoxic** The ability to poison genetic material, with a likely result of either cancer or damage to next generation.

**Job–years** A measure of work to perform a set task. A 100 job–year task might give 100 people work for one year or ten people work for ten years.

**Ischaemic heart disease (IHD)** A term that encompasses both angina (heart pain due to inadequate blood supply) and coronary thrombosis (heart attacks).

**Longitudinal studies** Studies that take a section of the population and study them as time passes.

**Meta-analysis** A method of reviewing the papers written about a subject, running together the statistics in order to obtain an overview of the results.

**Office of Population Censuses and Surveys (OPCS)** One of the British government's statistical departments.

**Panel (field) studies** Studies involving groups of volunteers who complete health diaries.

**Pathogens** Disease-causing organisms.

**Pavlovian psychology** A field of psychology which demonstrates the association between stimuli in the environment and responses in the organism.

**Standardized mortality rate (SMR)** A comparison of the death rate for a given population with the expected average for a wider population. An SMR of 100 is 'average'; 150 means a 50% increase, 200 means a doubling of the death rate and so on.

**Topography** Natural and artificial features of a locality; the 'lie of the land'.

**Trident–hour** A measurement of funding, equivalent to the amount of money spent each hour on the running costs of the pointless Trident nuclear 'deterrent' submarines; equivalent to £125 000 (official estimates) or £195 000 (Greenpeace estimates).

# Index

Note: Figures and Tables are indicated by italic page numbers.